GCSE History

Medicine through time

Second Edition

Aaron Wilkes

OXFORD
UNIVERSITY PRESS

OXFORD
UNIVERSITY PRESS

Great Clarendon Street, Oxford OX2 6DP

Oxford University Press is a department of the University of Oxford.
It furthers the University's objective of excellence in research,
scholarship, and education by publishing worldwide in

Oxford   New York

Auckland   Cape Town   Dar es Salaam   Hong Kong   Karachi
Kuala Lumpur   Madrid   Melbourne   Mexico City   Nairobi
New Delhi   Shanghai   Taipei   Toronto

With offices in

Argentina   Austria   Brazil   Chile   Czech Republic   France   Greece
Guatemala   Hungary   Italy   Japan   Poland   Portugal   Singapore
South Korea   Switzerland   Thailand   Turkey   Ukraine   Vietnam

Oxford is a registered trade mark of Oxford University Press
in the UK and in certain other countries

British Library Cataloguing in Publication Data

Data available

ISBN 978-1-85008-461-7

FD4617

10 9 8 7 6 5 4 3 2

Printed in Spain by Cayfosa Impresia Iberica

Paper used in the production of this book is a natural, recyclable product
made from wood grown in sustainable forests. The manufacturing process
conforms to the environmental regulations of the country of origin.

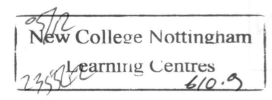
Acknowledgements

Aaron Wilkes hereby asserts his moral right to be identified as the author of this
work in accordance with the Copyright, Designs and Patents Act 1988.

Text design and layout: Neil Sutton, Pumpkin House

Illustrator(s): Celia Hart; Neil Sutton (p.10; p.48 [bottom]; p.49; p.56 [right];
p.64; p.104; p.132; pp.136–7; p.145; pp.162–3)

Cover design: Richard Jervis Design

Front cover image: Wellcome Library, London.

The author wishes to thank Kate Greig for her hard work and patience. He
would also like to acknowledge the help and support of Emma Wilkes during
the preparation of this book.

Text acknowledgements

p.15 www.mnsu.edu/emuseum/prehistory/egypt/dailylife/ medicine (top right);
p.19 *History of Medicine* by Tony Triggs, Collins Educational (1988); p.25
Herophilus: The Art of Medicine in Early Alexandria: Edition, Translation and Essays
by Herophilus, Cambridge University Press (1989); p.26 *History of Medicine* by
Tony Triggs, Collins Educational (1988); p.30 *History of Medicine* by Tony Triggs,
Collins Educational (1988); p.35 *History of Medicine* by Tony Triggs, Collins
Educational (1988); p.42 *Schools History Project: Medicine Through Time for OCR
GCSE* by Colin Shephard, Hodder Murray (2003); p.43 *Medicine & Health
Through Time: an SHP Development Study* by Ian Dawson, Ian Coulson, Hodder
Murray (1996); p.45 *Understanding History* by John Child, Paul Shuter, David
Taylor, Tim Hodge, Heinemann (1991); p.59 *History of Medicine* by Tony Triggs,
Collins Educational (1988); pp.62–3 BBC Bitesize; p.73 *Schools History Project:
Medicine Through Time for OCR GCSE* by Colin Shephard, Hodder Murray
(2003); p.76 *In Search of History: 1485–1714* by J.F. Aylett, Hodder Murray
(1984); pp.80–1 *Discovering the Past: Changing Role of Women (Discovering the
Past for GCSE)*, Hodder Murray (1996); pp.84–5 BBC Bitesize; p.118 *Explaining
Epidemics and other Studies in the History of Medicine* by Charles E. Rosenberg,
Cambridge University Press (1992); p.119 *Health and Medicine, 1750–1900*
(Longman Modern British History) by John Robottom, Longman (1991); p.131
Disease and its Control by Robert Hudson, Longman (1987); *History of Medicine*
by Tony Triggs, Collins Educational (1988); p.149 Based on the *Daily Mail*,
November (2006); pp.160–1 BBC Bitesize.

Photo acknowledgements

p.6 © Bettmann/Corbis; p.8–9 © Penny Tweedie/CORBIS; pp.16–7 MARY
EVANS/DOUGLAS MCCARTHY; p.17 Mary Evans Picture Library; p.22 © Corbis;
p.24 The Wellcome Trust; p.30 © Alan Copson/JAI/Corbis; p.36 The Wellcome
Trust; p.43 Museum of London; p.45 Edinburgh University Library; p.50 The
British Library, MS Sloane, 1977, fol 50.v. (left); p.50 © Bettmann/Corbis
(right); pp.52–3 © Corbis; p.54 Active Life, handwritten by Jean Henry, about
1482: AP-HP Musée; p.58 © Archivo Iconografico, S.A./CORBIS; p.60 AKG,
London (top); p.60 Getty Images (bottom); p.66 Bodleian Library; p.67 AKG,
London; p.69 © Bettmann/CORBIS (top); p.69 © Archivo Iconografico,
S.A./CORBIS (bottom); p.71 The Wellcome Trust (top); p.71 Fotomas Index
(bottom); p.72 © Bettmann/CORBIS; p.73 The Wellcome Trust; p.74 The
Wellcome Trust; p.75 Museum of London; p.76 © Bettmann/CORBIS; p.77
Fotomas Index; p.79 © Bettmann/CORBIS; p.82 AKG, London; p.83
Bayerisches National Museum; p.88 The Wellcome Trust; p.90 CORBIS; p.96
MARY EVANS/EXPLORER/WOLF; P.97 Getty Images; p.98 Mary Evans Picture
Library; p.100 The Wellcome Trust; p.101 © Hulton-Deutsch
Collection/CORBIS; p.103 The Wellcome Trust (top); p.103 © Michael
Nicholson/CORBIS (bottom); p.105 Mary Evans Picture Library; p.105 Hulton
Archive/Getty; p.108 Bridgeman Art Library/Royal College of Surgeons, UK;
p.109 The Wellcome Trust; p.110 The Wellcome Trust; p.111 The Wellcome
Trust; p.112 © Hulton-Deutsch Collection/CORBIS; p.113 The Wellcome Trust;
p.114 Art Directors; p.117 Mary Evans Picture Library; p.123 City of London,
London Metropolitan Archives; p.129 © Bettmann/CORBIS; p.130 ©
Bettmann/CORBIS; p.141 Mary Evans Picture Library (both); p.142 © PASCAL
ROSSIGNOL/Reuters/CORBIS (left); p.142 © Roland Quadrini/Reuters/CORBIS
(right); p.143 © Lester Lefkowitz/CORBIS (top); p.143 © Bettmann/CORBIS
(bottom); p.146 Pictorial Press Ltd/Alamy (top left); p. 146 Rex Features (top
right); p.146 Trinity Mirror/Mirrorpix/Alamy (bottom right); p.147 Mary Evans
Picture Library/Onslows Auctions Limited (top); p.147 Mary Evans Picture
Library/Illustrated London News (right); p.147 Hulton-Deutsch
Collection/CORBIS (middle); p.147 Corbis (bottom); p.152 Aaron Wilkes; p.153
© Tim Matheson/MaXx Images Inc./zefa/CORBIS; p.160 Bridgeman Art
Library/Royal College of Surgeons, UK (top); p.160 The Wellcome Trust
(bottom).

Contents

Medicine through time: an introduction

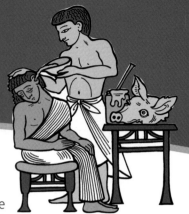

The human body is an amazing machine. Underneath your skin, there are hundreds of muscles and bones, thousands of miles of tubes, millions of nerves and billions of cells. Long ago, people didn't know how our bodies worked. This led to many weird and wonderful treatments when people were ill. Today, we still don't know exactly how our bodies work – and still there are many weird and wonderful treatments out there to try!

The story of medicine and health from 'long ago' to modern times is a fascinating journey. To help make sense of it all, your journey in this book has been divided into the following periods:

- medicine in prehistoric times – so far back that there are no written records!;
- medicine in the ancient world – delve into the world of Ancient Egyptians, Greeks and Romans;
- medicine in the Middle Ages – study why very little medical progress was made;
- the Medical Renaissance – investigate what new discoveries were made … and what impact they had;
- medicine in the eighteenth and nineteenth centuries – how was the true cause of disease found?;
- medicine and health since 1900 – what progress has been made over the last 100 years … and what does the future hold?

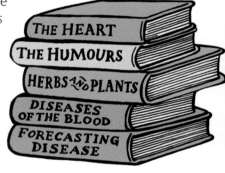

You will also investigate what people thought *caused* disease and illness in various periods of history.

For example, you will study that :

- evil spirits got the blame for most illnesses in the ancient world … as well as your 'humours' being out of balance!;
- the position of the planets was pinpointed as a major cause of disease during the Middle Ages … or having too much blood in your body;

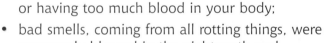
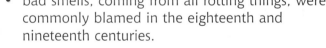

- bad smells, coming from all rotting things, were commonly blamed in the eighteenth and nineteenth centuries.

This book will help you to investigate how people in different periods of time used different methods to *treat* illness. For example, you will discover that :

- for thousands of years, people treated headaches by getting someone to drill a hole in their head!
- a common cure for plague was to shave a chicken's bottom and tie it under their arm;
- pupils at one English school were once *encouraged* to start smoking to fend off a killer disease;
- modern analysis of some of the oldest – and most curious – herbal remedies has shown that they would have actually worked because the herbs used contain ingredients *still* used in medicine today.

FACT *The world's biggest ever killer!*

Half the human beings who have *ever* died, perhaps as many as 50 billion people, have been killed by female mosquitoes (the males only bite plants!). Mosquitoes carry more than 100 potentially killer diseases including malaria, yellow fever, elephantiasis and dengue fever. Even today, mosquitoes kill one person every 12 seconds.

For example, heart monitors can now transfer details of a beating heart directly to a computer via a satellite link. This means the patient can recover at home rather than in a hospital ward and, as a result, more hospital beds are made available.

Whilst studying health and medicine, you will be asked to consider some very important questions. The questions will appear time and time again and by the end of your studies, you *should* have developed your own ideas and examples in answer to these questions.

You will be asked to think about:

- how medicine has changed;
- how factors such as war, religion, science and technology, individual brilliance, good luck and government action have brought about changes in medicine;
- how fast change happened – and if change has always brought benefits;
- why people had different ideas about what caused disease;
- what different ideas people had about how to cure illness.

Before you start your studies, can you think of any ways that the factors listed might cause change in medicine? Think carefully. It is a more straightforward question than you might think.

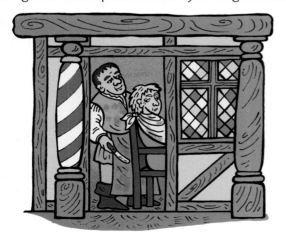

WORK

1. **a** Make a note of at least three times you or a member of your family has been ill, injured, suffered from a disease or has needed medical care. For each one, write down all the people involved in getting you or them better. Also note down the treatments and methods used.

   b Now circle anything that you think happened 100 years ago. For example, if you broke your leg playing football, were taken by ambulance to hospital, seen by a doctor, X-rayed, put in a cast and given crutches – do you think all the people involved and the treatment you received happened 100 years ago?

   c Underline anything you think would have happened 1000 years ago.

2. Think about the following factors that have caused changes in medicine:
   - war
   - religion
   - science and technology
   - individual brilliance
   - good luck
   - government action.

   Can you think of at least one way each of the factors might affect medicine in any way? For example, 'When countries fight wars, they have to put a lot of resources into new types of surgery so that injured soldiers can get back to fighting as soon as possible – so war speeds up the development of surgery.'

Why has he got a hole in his head?

Look at **Source A**. Even the least observant person will notice the big hole in the side of this skull. Modern experts know that the hole wasn't drilled after the person had died – it was made whilst they were still alive … we know they survived because the bone at the edge of the hole had begun to grow again! So why did this person have a hole cut through the side of their head? At what time in history did this operation take place? And what does this rather scary operation tell us about health, medicine and beliefs at that time?

Source A ▾ _The operation to remove the circular piece of skull or to drill through the head was known as **trepanning**._

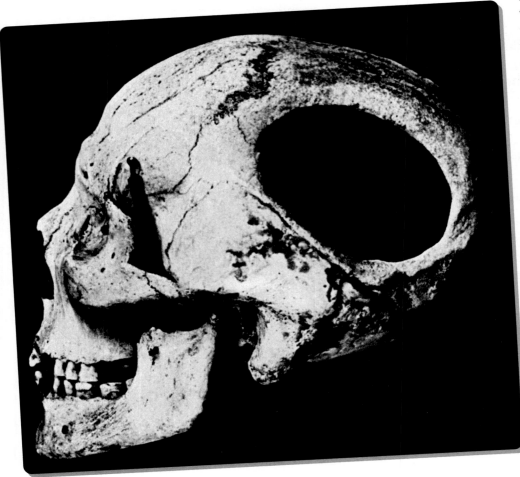

The skull pictured in **Source A** dates back to **prehistoric** times.

Prehistoric means 'before we had written records' so to understand the times, we depend on other types of evidence, such as the tools people used, the cave paintings they drew and the actual bones of the people themselves. In fact, when looking at health and medicine in prehistoric times, bones are our biggest clues as to what people thought and did about medical problems.

Although people capable of making tools have lived on earth for about 2½ million years, most of our evidence comes from bones we have discovered that are between 10 000 and 20 000 years old. These people were hunter-gatherers, living in small groups and moving around the country, looking for good shelter and food supplies. Life for them must have been very tough … and usually short!

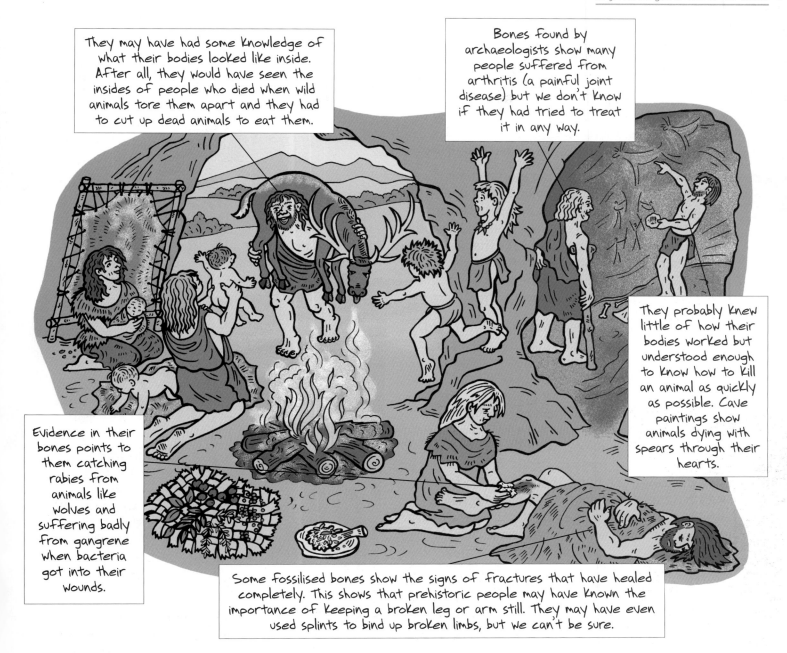

They may have had some knowledge of what their bodies looked like inside. After all, they would have seen the insides of people who died when wild animals tore them apart and they had to cut up dead animals to eat them.

Bones found by archaeologists show many people suffered from arthritis (a painful joint disease) but we don't know if they had tried to treat it in any way.

Evidence in their bones points to them catching rabies from animals like wolves and suffering badly from gangrene when bacteria got into their wounds.

They probably knew little of how their bodies worked but understood enough to know how to kill an animal as quickly as possible. Cave paintings show animals dying with spears through their hearts.

Some fossilised bones show the signs of fractures that have healed completely. This shows that prehistoric people may have known the importance of keeping a broken leg or arm still. They may have even used splints to bind up broken limbs, but we can't be sure.

On a more positive note, prehistoric men and women wouldn't have suffered from some of the diseases that are common in the modern world.

- They must have eaten a lot of wild plants and berries that would have kept them healthy.
- They would not have contracted any of the diseases and illnesses associated with eating 'fast food', smoking or drinking alcohol.
- As they only lived in one place for a short period of time, they didn't pollute their water supplies and pile up human waste and filth that could attract disease-carrying insects.

FACT *And you let him lick your face!*

As prehistoric people began to settle in one place, they began to farm. There is evidence that they kept dogs, cattle, pigs, sheep and chickens. Disease from these animals would have spread to humans, for example, experts have estimated that humans share over 60 diseases with dogs and nearly 50 with cattle and poultry.

Source B is a copy of a picture found in a cave in Southern France. It shows a man dressed up like a wild stag. Most archaeologists think that the man was a **witch doctor**, which suggests that prehistoric people blamed evil spirits for diseases they didn't fully understand. They probably thought that strangely dressed tribesmen (or paintings of them) would frighten away the evil spirits that caused their illnesses.

Prehistoric people knew that the most common cause of pain was an injury, but sometimes people suffered pain without showing any signs of injury. Perhaps they wondered what was entering their bodies and hurting them without leaving a mark! The idea of an 'evil spirit' seemed an obvious answer.

So what about that hole in the head?

Prehistoric people believed that evil spirits could live in a person's head and cause them pain. In order to release them, they needed to remove a piece of skull. Using a sharp piece of flint or basic drill, a hole was made or part of the skull was chipped away. Amazingly, many people must have survived this ordeal because skulls have been found with holes that had almost closed again, proving that they had lived for many years after the operation. Also, the bits of bone removed from skulls have also been found, usually with a hole through the middle, suggesting that they may have been worn round the neck as a lucky charm.

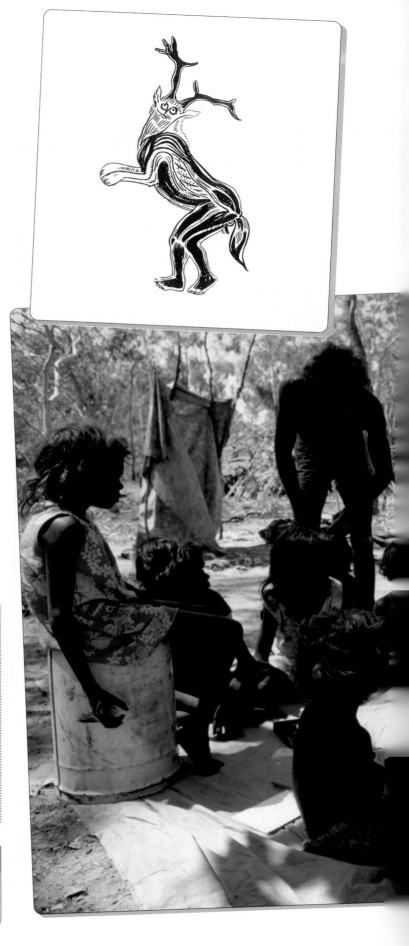

FACT *Prehistoric medicine today*

In parts of Australia, there are Aborigines whose way of life and beliefs have not changed for centuries. From them, we can discover a lot about prehistoric medicine. For example, we know that their beliefs are usually superstitious and magical. Often, they use witch doctors to treat their diseases and curse their enemies. They also use herbs to cure illnesses. Indeed, in some parts of South America, where tribes still live a 'primitive' life, scientists are desperately trying to find out more about cures before jungle clearance causes rare plants and ancient ways of life to die out.

TOP EXAM TIP

For your exam make sure you understand that prehistoric and Aboriginal medicine is based on supernatural thinking.

◄ **Source B** *A picture of a witch doctor found in a cave in Southern France.*

WISE UP WORDS

- trepanning   prehistoric   witch doctor

Source C ▼ *A health visitor talking to Aborigines in Australia. They are discussing how effective some herbal remedies can be.*

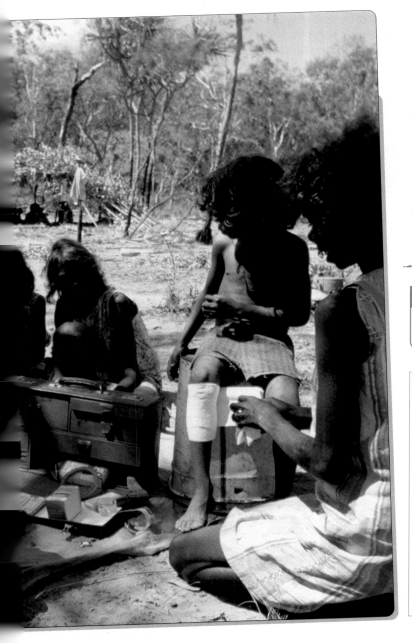

WORK

1 Write a sentence or two to explain what is meant by the following:
   - prehistoric
   - witch doctor
   - trepanning.

2 We know very little about what prehistoric people thought about medicine. Why is it impossible to be sure about how they treated the sick and wounded?

3 Look at the cartoon on page 7.
   a What evidence is there that prehistoric people cared for those who were injured?
   b Prehistoric people probably knew little about anatomy (how the body is made up inside). What opportunities did they have to learn about this?

4 Look at **Sources A** and **B**.
   a How do these sources help us to understand how prehistoric people explained illness?
   b How do these sources help us to understand how prehistoric people treated illness?

5 Why did prehistoric people not suffer from some of the diseases common today? Explain your answer carefully.

CLASSIC EXAM QUESTION

Outline what prehistoric people believed about the cause and cure of illness.

SUMMARY

- Prehistoric Britons believed that the spirits caused illness and disease.

- They were able to treat simple surface wounds and there was much use of herbs and plants. Evidence shows that trepanning was used.

- Medicine men provided medical care, but women were closely involved in treating illnesses as wives and mothers.

What sort of learner are you?

Lots of recent research has suggested that people learn in different ways – in other words, all of us have a **preferred learning style**. Although there are lots of different ways to learn, in recent years experts have narrowed it down to three key styles: Visual, Auditory and Kinaesthetic (VAK). In many schools today, teachers have worked hard to make students aware of their preferred learning style – and it is fairly easy to go online, answer a few short questions and work out whether you are mainly a visual, auditory or kinaesthetic learner. However, for those students who have no idea what their preferred learning style is, the chart below may help you out.

Do you like...?	Possible preferred learning style	
Seeing, reading, learning by looking at diagrams, demonstrations, displays, handouts, films, charts etc., using highlighters to colour-code	Visual	
Listening, speaking, learning by copying down information from DVDs, podcasts or TV, discussing things with friends after just learning them, saying things over and over again until they 'sink in'	Auditory	
Touching, doing, learning by creating imaginative charts, grids and timelines, re-enacting situations, cutting things up and rearranging them on the page, visits for understanding	Kinaesthetic	

Knowing your preferred learning style will help you revise for your exams. It should help you focus your revision in a way most suited to help you learn and retain the most information.

Look carefully at the targeted revision techniques detailed on these pages. Once you have worked out your preferred learning style, try to use some of the techniques when revising.

Top tips

Don't use just the one revision style to get your
brain really buzzing, use a variety of techniques.

*If you are a **visual** learner...*

- Try to put your notes into particular categories.
- Organise your notes in to sections – try colour coding them – perhaps write the key facts in a bold colour.
- Draw pictures or find photos from the internet to accompany your notes
- Write the things you need to remember on wall charts and on posters to hang around your bedroom.
- It will help you if memorise various parts of your note-taking.
- Use colour-coded index cards to help you to organise your revision by concentrating on one colour set each night.
- Use video clips to help you remember the facts you need to know, making notes as you watch.

*If you are an **auditory** learner...*

- Very often it is important to discuss your revision with your friends, talk about the things you have just learned and understand.
- It is easier sometimes to do your homework with other students who are also auditory learners.
- Record your own revision onto tape or your iPod and play it back to yourself.
- It is important to say information over and over in order to retain it.
- If possible act out or tell a story about various things you need to remember from your studies. You will then be able to imagine the story you have created in your head when writing it down in an exam.
- Sometimes it could help to try to make up a rhyme about what you are trying to remember, you could also try to put it to a tune.
- Try studying in a group, this might help you to learn.
- Use background music to help you concentrate.

*If you are a **kinaesthetic** learner...*

- Copy things out over and over again making them neat and presented in an organised fashion.
- Visit as many places linked to your studies as possible.
- Wherever possible try to trace the key words you need to remember with your hand or finger.
- Try to construct things whilst you are studying e.g. a model to help you learn.
- Create flash cards to help prompt you when learning.
- Take frequent breaks when you are studying.
- Use memory techniques using hand gestures to help you to remember.
- Don't read large amounts of text at any one time – you will not take 50% of it in.

What's so special about Ancient Egypt?

> Understand what the various factors were in Ancient Egypt that affected health and medicine.

About 5000 years ago, one of the first (and most famous) great civilisations lived on the banks of the River Nile in Egypt. Every autumn, the River Nile overflowed its banks and the water and mud made the land on either side of the River extremely good for growing crops. The Egyptian farmers were so successful that they became rich … very, very rich! There was plenty of work for jewellers, house builders, doctors, shopkeepers, merchants and tomb builders too. Indeed, Egypt was one of the wealthiest countries the world had ever known, with powerful rulers, large cities and thriving businesses. But what factors about life in Ancient Egypt affected medicine?

Money

Rich people paid doctors to look after them. The king (or pharaoh) employed a whole team of doctors. But Egyptian law made sure that even the poorest people could have a doctor's help if they needed it. Egypt's wealth meant that the country had many specialist craftsmen to make fine jewellery or ornaments. They also made fine bronze medical instruments for the doctors to work with, meaning they had better equipment to work with than doctors from earlier times.

The Nile

The River Nile itself gave Egyptian doctors a theory about how disease was caused. The Egyptians had built a system of channels and ditches to direct water from the Nile to surrounding fields. If a waterway became blocked, the fields would dry out and crops would die. Egyptian doctors applied this knowledge to their patients. They knew that the human body had lots of channels too, carrying blood, air and food. They decided that disease was caused when these vessels became blocked. As a result, they examined their patients very carefully, looking for lumps or any other explanation for a blockage. This led to treatment like **bloodletting** or the use of **laxatives** to clear any possible signs of a blockage.

TOP EXAM TIP

Make sure you can work out how each of these 5 key factors shown on these pages could affect the discovery of medical knowledge.

Writing

The Egyptians developed **papyrus**, a kind of paper made from reeds. They also used a system of writing, using symbols called **hieroglyphics**. This meant they could keep records of illnesses and treatments and this knowledge could be added to over time and preserved for later generations of doctors.

Trade

Egyptian merchants traded with others from India, China and Africa. New herbs and plants arrived in Egypt, allowing healers to use a wide variety of herbal medicines.

Religion

Egyptian religious beliefs may have helped doctors to learn more about the human body. Egyptians believed that there was life after death and people needed their body and their vital organs when they passed into the afterlife. As a result, they went to great lengths to preserve or **mummify** bodies. The liver, lungs, stomach, intestines and brain were taken out, placed in jars and soaked in a preservative solution. The body itself was soaked in salts and wrapped in bandages to stop it decaying. The people who did this must have learned about the body's vital organs but may not have understood the proper roles of the parts of the body.

WISE UP WORDS

bloodletting   laxatives   papyrus hieroglyphics   mummification

WORK

1 **a** Most Egyptians believed, like prehistoric people, that evil spirits caused illness. But there was also a theory that blocked channels caused disease. Briefly explain why you think they believed in the 'blocked channel theory'.

b How did their belief in the 'blocked channel theory' influence the way some patients were treated?

2 **a** Make brief notes to explain how each of the following factors of Egyptian life affected English medicine:
- money
- trade
- the Nile
- writing
- religion.

NOTE: As a challenge, try to keep your notes on each factor limited to two sentences.

b Choose one of the factors that you think was particularly important and write a paragraph to explain your choice.

'Doctor, doctor...!'

Topic Focus

▸ In this topic you will consider how Egyptian doctors worked, what the Egyptians believed about the cause of illness, and how natural and supernatural ideas worked together.

The Egyptians believed that disease and death were caused by an angry god or an evil spirit. At medical schools, attached to temples, doctors learned to drive out the evil spirits using magic rituals, lucky charms or special potions. In fact, the duties of Egyptian doctors were wide-ranging – they set broken bones, fixed teeth and performed small operations – and some had individual titles like 'the palace eye doctor' or 'the one who understands the internal fluids' and even 'the guardian of the anus'!

The Egyptians suffered from many of the illnesses and injuries still common today. A great deal of our knowledge comes from ancient manuscripts that show treatments for eye infections, measles, tuberculosis, toothache, malaria, broken bones and breathing problems. These documents contain recipes and spells for all sorts of ailments. They recommend a variety of substances to use, including plants, minerals and the droppings, blood, brains and urine of a number of animals. One document – the *Kahun Papyrus* as it is known – is a text that focuses mainly on women and childbirth. It deals with such topics as the reproductive system, conception, testing for pregnancy, childbirth itself and contraception. Amongst the substances prescribed for contraception are crocodile dung, honey and sour milk!

Look through the following sources very carefully. They will allow you to build up a picture of how the Egyptians treated illness and injury.

Source A ▾ *Based on the* Ebers Papyrus, *an Egyptian document dating from the sixteenth century.*

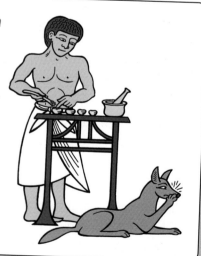

For indigestion

Crush a dog's tooth and put it inside four sugar cakes. Eat for four days.

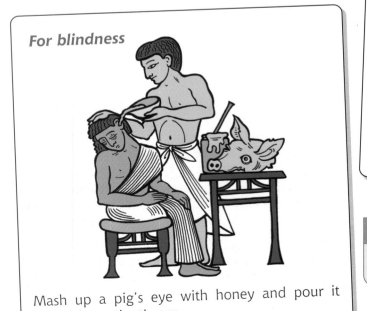

For blindness

Mash up a pig's eye with honey and pour it down the patient's ear.

TOP EXAM TIP

Make sure you know the difference between NATURAL and SUPERNATURAL ideas.

For lesions (wounds) of the skin

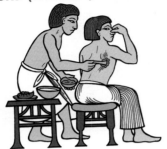

After the scab has fallen off, put on it a scribe's (a man who writes letters) excrement mixed with fresh milk. Rub into the skin.

Cure for burns

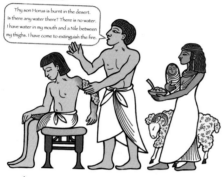

'Thy son Horus is burnt in the desert. Is there any water there? There is no water. I have water in my mouth and a Nile between my thighs. I have come to extinguish the fire.'

Create a mixture of breast milk from a woman who has had a male child, gum and sheep's hair. Whilst rubbing the mixture into the burns, say: 'Thy son Horus is burnt in the desert. Is there any water there? There is no water. I have water in my mouth and a Nile between my thighs. I have come to extinguish the fire.'

Source B ▼ From the Edwin Smith Papyrus, a collection of medical treatments, recipes and spells written around 1600BC. There are 48 cases of surgery in the Edwin Smith Papyrus, each with a careful description of examination, symptoms, diagnosis and treatment – very similar to what a doctor does today.

For treating a broken nose

Examination: Examine a man with a bleeding nose, part of it squashed, disfigured or swollen.

Diagnosis: You should say, 'Should have a broken nose and I can treat this'.

Treatment: Clean the nose with two plugs of linen. Put two plugs soaked in grease into his nostrils. Tell him to rest until the swelling goes down, bandage his nose and treat him every day until he recovers.

Source C ▼ From a website. The source shows how the Egyptians used natural cures (eating well, regular bathing, herbal remedies) side by side with supernatural ideas like praying to their gods.

"The instructions for a healthy life included much bathing, and often shaving one's head and body hair, and maintaining their dietary restrictions against raw fish and other animals considered unclean to eat. Also, and in addition to a purified lifestyle, it was not uncommon for the Egyptians to undergo dream analysis to find a cure or cause for illness, as well as to ask for a priest to aid them with magic. This obviously portrays that religious magical rites were intertwined in the healing process as well as in creating a proper lifestyle."

FACT *My God!*

According to the Egyptians, their gods controlled everything, including the movement of the stars and the flooding of the Nile. They turned to them to explain illnesses and provide cures too. Gods, included Seth, who brought disease by sending demons to enter the body whilst Osiris, Thoth and Horus could heal you. Bes protected pregnant women. Temples and shrines were built to worship these gods.

WORK

1 Imagine you are an Egyptian doctor in Ancient Egypt. Write a diary for a few days showing what complaints patients came to you with, how you examined them and what treatments you used.

2 Look at **Source B**. According to this source, Egyptian doctors were developing sensible, intelligent cures for some injuries. So why do you think they still used some of the treatments described in **Source A**?

3 From what you have read so far, do you think the Ancient Egyptians were more or less advanced in medicine than prehistoric people? Give reasons for your answer.

The Mummy Maker

Topic Focus

▶ This topic will consider how and why Ancient Egyptians carried out the mummification process.

Ancient Egypt is famous for its 'mummies'. Mummification, as the process is known, was a complicated process carried out by specialists called **embalmers**. The most well-known of all was the royal embalmer – personal servant to the kings of Egypt. An interview with him may have gone something like this:

So why were people turned into mummies?

We believe that people have a life after death and that you need your body in the afterlife. You need to preserve the body properly or it will be of no use to you as a rotten mess!

How do you stop the bodies from rotting?

We have to do this very quickly as these bodies rot fast in the hot weather. First, we pull out the brain through the nose and rinse out the skull with chemicals. Next, we cut along the side of the body with a sharp stone and remove the intestines, stomach, lungs, heart and liver.

What happens next?

The heart is rinsed in chemicals and placed back inside the body. The heart is so important, you see, as blood flows from the heart to every part of the body. The other organs are sealed in jars under the protection of the god Horus until the dead person needs them.

And the rest of the body?

The body itself is washed in a solution of palm wine, milk, spices and oil. Then a covering of salt is rubbed in and left for 40 days.

Why 40 days?

Forty is a magical number to us ... and it's also about how long the salt takes to dry out the body. Then the skin is softened by rubbing it with oil before being wrapped in fine linen bandages.

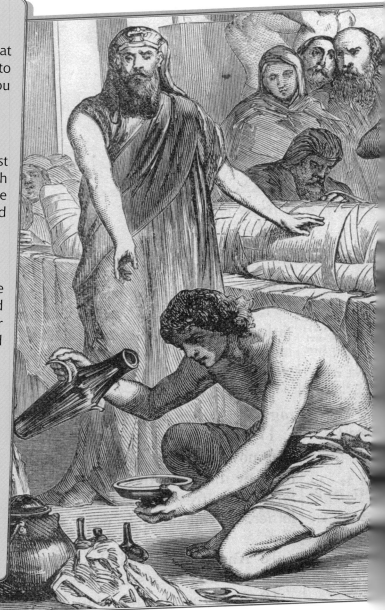

What about burial?

The 'mummy' is then placed in a coffin – some coffins are quite beautiful, especially royal ones – and given to the priests for burial. The jar of organs will go to the burial chamber too.

And do you feel you're an expert on the human body?

I know a bit about the human body but we don't really know exactly how each body part works. That's for the gods to know I suppose. And we're not allowed to cut up the body into small pieces either – dissection is banned – people need all of their body intact for the afterlife.

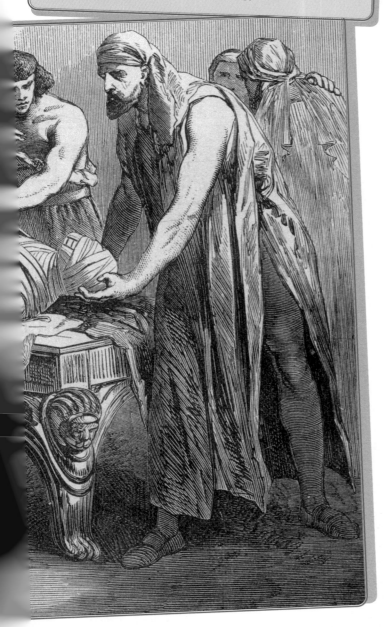

Source A ▼ *The head of the mummy of Rameses III.*

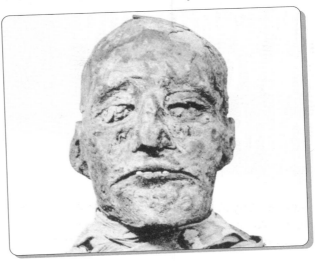

WISE UP WORD

- embalmers

WORK

1 If Egyptians wanted to know more about parts of the body, how did the mummification process:
   i) help them?   ii) hinder them?
2 Based on your studies of medicine in Ancient Egypt, copy and complete the following chart:

Who treated the sick?

What did they know (or not know) about the human body?

Egyptian medicine

What did they think caused disease?

What methods were used to prevent or treat illness?

CLASSIC EXAM QUESTION

What knowledge of anatomy and surgery was there in Ancient Egypt?

ii) Ancient Greece

So what did the Greeks think?

Topic Focus

➤ This double page will outline what part religion played when the Ancient Greeks looked for cures for their illnesses.

The Ancient Greeks (those who lived in Greece over 2000 years ago) play a very important part in the story of health and medicine. Their new ideas about the causes of illness – and their methods of treatment – remained important for many centuries.

The Greeks believed that illness was a punishment sent by the gods. They prayed to these gods for a cure. Special healing temples – called **Asclepeia** – were found all over the Greek world. A single temple was called an Asclepion. They were named after a doctor called Asclepius, whom many people had come to regard as a god because he was so famous and so popular.

So what was an Asclepion like?

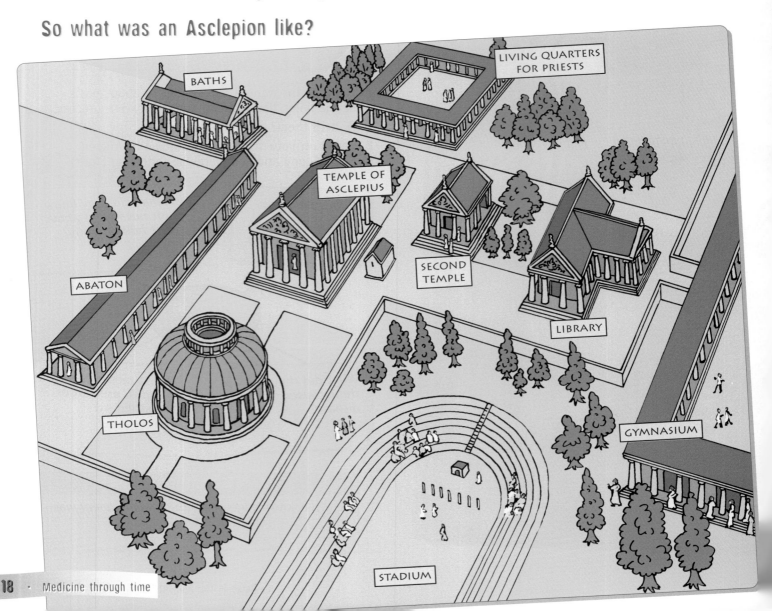

BATHS

LIVING QUARTERS FOR PRIESTS

TEMPLE OF ASCLEPIUS

SECOND TEMPLE

LIBRARY

ABATON

THOLOS

GYMNASIUM

STADIUM

When a patient first arrived for their 'treatment', they would sacrifice an animal in front of a huge statue of Asclepius. In the 'tholos', they would then wash in water rich in salts and minerals, hoping that the gods would wash away all the guilt and evil inside them. This would last several days.

When a priest decided a patient was ready, he or she was led into the temple to pray before being taken to the 'abaton' to sleep on beds covered with the skins of animals sacrificed to the gods. Here they slept whilst snakes (a sacred reptile to the Greeks) were allowed to slide across their bodies and touch them with their flickering tongues! Some woke up feeling a lot better whilst others, who still said they were ill, were told to return when their faith in the gods was a little stronger!

Source A ▾ *From* History of Medicine.

"We know about the temples because the ruins still exist today, and some of the tablets describing cures can still be read. According to one tablet:

'Euippos has had for six years the point of a spear in his cheek. As he was sleeping, the god extracted the spear head and put it in his hands.'

We also know about the temples from ancient books and plays. One play describes how a blind man was cured by two huge snakes which licked his eyelids during the night."

So why were so many patients cured?

Few people today believe in the Greek gods and the healing powers of snakes but there is little doubt that many people were actually cured in these temples. There are several explanations:

• The power of positive thinking – the patient actually believed they could be cured. Today, doctors accept that if a patient believes a certain form of treatment will work, they will worry less about their health and start to feel better.

• Good habits – when the patients entered these peaceful temples, they forgot their daily routine and troubles. Instead, they settled for peace and quiet, a good diet and plenty of restful massage (some people stayed for months!). It is little wonder that patients suffering from headaches, sleeplessness or indigestion soon felt better!

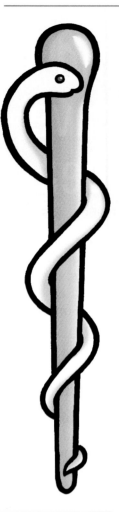

Source B ▸ *You will see this symbol on ambulances and paramedics' uniforms throughout the world. A sacred snake and the staff of the god Asclepius have survived as symbols of health and medicine for thousands of years.*

WISE UP WORD
• Asclepeia

WORK

1 Look at the different buildings in the temple complex. All were useful in health care. For each building, explain how it might have made a patient healthier.

2 Large pits have been found at some of the temple sites. What do you think these pits were for?

3 'Asclepeia were only about treating patients by supernatural methods.' Explain whether you agree or disagree with this statement.

CLASSIC EXAM QUESTION
Describe what happened at an Asclepia.

Did the Greeks have any new ideas?

Topic Focus

▸ What was the theory of the four humours?
▸ How did knowledge of this influence doctors in their work?

Exam Focus

▸ You must make sure you know about the theory of the four humours: take the time to prepare for this in the exam.

The Greeks believed that illness was a punishment sent by the gods to whom they prayed for a cure. But Greek thinkers were very interested in science too. They weren't satisfied believing that gods controlled everything. They wanted more rational explanations of how and why things worked. They began to think that diseases could actually have natural causes … and as a result, there might be such a thing as a natural cure. Some Greek thinkers went so far as saying that a patient's belief in magic and the gods could actually prevent effective medical treatment!

So what were these new 'natural' ideas about illness and cure?

The theory of the four humours

Greek thinkers thought that everything in the world was made up of four basic elements – earth, air, water and fire. Each of these elements had certain characteristics – earth is cold and dry, air is hot and wet, water is cold and wet, and fire is hot and dry. The Greeks linked these characteristics to four liquids they believed were contained in a person's body.

These four liquids, or humours as they called them, were black bile, blood, phlegm and yellow bile. They said that black bile is cold and dry, blood is hot and wet, phlegm is cold and wet and yellow bile is hot and dry. They went so far as to link seasons of the year to these humours too (see **Source A**).

Source A ▾ *A chart showing the links between the humours and the elements. Interestingly, historians still didn't know what black bile actually was!*

When the humours were in balance in a person's body, they were considered healthy. However, when this balance was upset (if there was too much of one humour and not enough of another), the result was illness (see **Source B**).

Source B ▾ *Greek doctor Hippocrates in* On the Constitution of Man *(c.500BC).*

> "Man's body has blood, phlegm, yellow bile and black bile. These make up his body and through them he feels illness or enjoys health. When all the humours are properly balanced and mingled, he feels the most perfect health. Illness occurs when one of the humours is in excess, or is reduced in amount, or is entirely missing from the body."

Element	Characteristics	Season	Humour
Earth	Cold and dry	Autumn	Black bile
Air	Hot and wet	Spring	Blood
Water	Cold and wet	Winter	Phlegm
Fire	Hot and dry	Summer	Yellow bile

TOP EXAM TIP

It is VITAL that you understand the theory of the four humours – spend your own time learning this famous theory.

In practical terms, a visit to a doctor might go like the cartoon in **Source C**.

Source C ▾ *Doctors visiting a patient in Ancient Greece.*

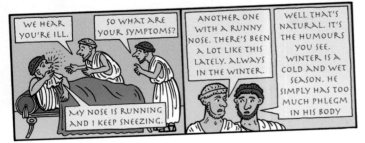

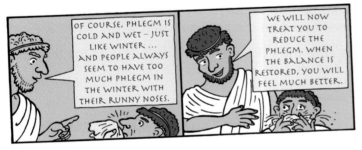

So how would a Greek doctor treat you?

The doctors didn't believe in interfering too much in order to put the humours back in balance. They thought that nature would balance them eventually and the job of a doctor was to help nature along.

If they concluded that you had too much blood in your body, they might cut you to let some of the blood out (known as bloodletting). They may encourage you to vomit or give you laxatives to 'clean out' your system.

Above all, they encouraged a 'balanced' lifestyle – a sensible amount of sleep, exercise, bathing and even sex! Their philosophy was very much one of 'prevention rather than cure'. In other words, doctors felt that a healthy balance to everything would lead to a healthy life. This is a belief we still hold today.

Source D ▾ *From* A Programme of Health, *an ancient Greek book. Note how the theory of good health is all about balance. Patients in summer, a hot and dry season, are advised to do things to make them cold and wet.*

"In summer, a person should drink more and eat less. This will keep the body cold and wet. Walking should be slow in summer too, to keep the body colder."

Source E ▾ *From the Greek doctor, Diocles. Very sensible advice indeed, don't you think?*

"Keeping healthy begins with the moment a man wakes up. After awakening, he should not arise at once but should wait until the heaviness of sleep has gone. After arising, he should rub oil over his body. Every day, he should wash his face and eyes using pure water. He should rub his teeth using peppermint powder and clean away the remnants of food. He should put perfumed oil on his nose and ears and wash his hair and comb it.

A young or middle-aged man should take a walk too. Long walks before meals clear out the body, prepare it for receiving food and give it more power for digesting."

WISE UP WORD

- theory of the four humours

WORK

1 **a** Make your own version of **Source A** using your own words, pictures and symbols.

   b Why do you think the Greeks believed in the theory of the four humours?

2 How did Greek doctors treat illness?

3 Look at **Source D**. In what ways is this advice based on the theory of the four humours?

4 Look at **Source E**. List the ways in which this advice would help someone to improve their health.

Hippocrates – the greatest doctor of all?

Topic Focus

This topic looks at:
▶ Who Hippocrates was and why he is important.
▶ His theories and his method of observation.

Almost 2500 years ago, a Greek doctor named Hippocrates began to question the old superstitious ideas about health and medicine that had been based on the gods and spirits.

His groundbreaking ideas for treating illness and looking after the sick were closely followed by the doctors of his time – and have influenced doctors from his day right up to the present.

So what was so special about Hippocrates?

Source A ▾ *The statue of Hippocrates (c.460–370BC), the ancient Greek doctor and philosopher.*

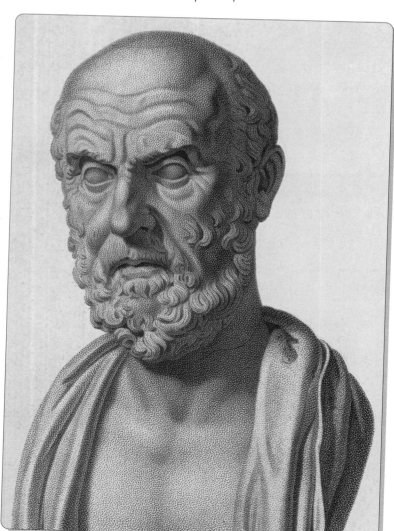

His ideas for treating patients

Hippocrates insisted that patients must be carefully observed and the findings recorded. The emphasis was on studying the patient and their lifestyle – their diet, work, exercise, sleep and environment – rather than the disease.

He felt doctors should:

- ask the patient about their symptoms;
- examine the patient carefully – listen to their breathing, take their pulse, examine the body and so on;
- ignore nothing;
- make a note of everything.

Only after careful observation should the appropriate drugs be selected and, as a last resort, an operation carried out if the chances of success were good (see **Sources B** and **C**).

Source B ▾ *Hippocrates' On Behaviour, 500BC.*

"A doctor must be able to remember all the drugs and their uses. You must get your medicine ready in good time. You must visit your patients often and be careful when you examine them. When you enter a patient's room, be calm and remember your bedside manners. Sometimes the patient may need telling off, sometimes comforting."

Source C ▾ *From* Hippocratic Writings: Epidemics.

Day 1: Fever, pain in his head and then became deaf. No sleep, bad fever, tongue dry.

Day 2: Delirious.

Day 6: Symptoms became worse.

Day 11: Constipated. Urine thick and coloured with substances scattered throughout.

Day 17: Swellings about both ears. Legs painful. No sleep.

Day 31: Diarrhoea with large discharges of watery matters. Urine thick. Swelling around ears gone.

His books

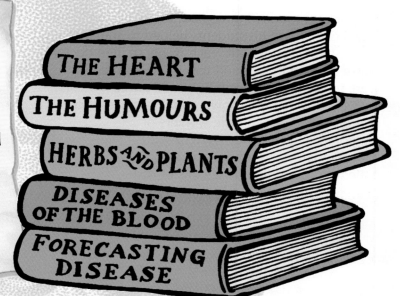

THE HEART
THE HUMOURS
HERBS AND PLANTS
DISEASES OF THE BLOOD
FORECASTING DISEASE

His theories

Hippocrates encouraged doctors to look for natural treatments rather than going to the gods for help. For example, he contradicted the view that epileptic fits were due to a god or evil spirit taking over the sufferer's brain (see **Source D**).

He also said that these, the natural causes of illness, included poor diet, unhealthy living conditions and weaknesses that are present at birth. He formulated a theory based on the humours to explain the cause of disease and treat it. Today, we know this theory was wrong but the main idea associated with it – that a patient should lead a balanced lifestyle – is one that stays with us today.

Source D ▾ *Hippocrates.*

"Epilepsy is not, in my view, any more sacred or divine than any other disease. Its supposed origin with the gods is due to man's inexperience and to their wonder at its peculiar character. Each disease has a natural cause … if we can find the cause, we can find the cure."

The *Hippocratic Collection* is a selection of books that doctors have used for years. Hippocrates wrote some of the books but not all; they have just come to be named after him. The books though present a huge step forward in medicine. It is the first detailed record of the ways in which different illnesses develop. They helped doctors for centuries to decide what an illness was and what would be a suitable treatment (see **Source E**).

Source E ▾ *From the* Hippocratic Collection.

"It is an excellent thing for a doctor to forecast. If he knows what the next symptoms are likely to be, he can give the patient the right treatment."

Source F ▾ *From the* Hippocratic Collection.

"If the pain is under the diaphragm, clear the bowels with a medicine made from black hellebore [a herb], cumin or other fragrant herbs. A bath will help **pneumonia** as it soothes pain and brings up the phlegm."

His legacy

Hippocrates founded a medical school on the Greek island of Kos and his students helped to spread his ideas. Before setting out, each newly trained doctor swore an oath that bound him to do his medical work to the best of his ability (see **Source G**). This oath is still very well known today. It makes it clear that doctors aren't miracle workers or magicians and that they have to keep high standards and work to benefit their patients – rather than make lots of cash!

Source G ▼ *The Hippocratic Oath.*

" I swear by Apollo, Asclepius and by all gods, that I will keep this oath. I will use treatment to help the sick to the best of my ability and judgement but never with a view to injury or wrongdoing. I will not give poison to anybody. I will be pure and holy in my life and practice. I will keep secret anything I see or hear professionally which ought not to be told."

Hippocrates advised that operations should only be carried out if the patient stood a good chance of survival. Greek doctors developed good techniques for setting broken bones and surgeons (the Hippocratic Oath said that doctors shouldn't use 'the knife, but will leave this to those men who do this work') performed some successful amputations. There is no evidence that Greek surgeons successfully operated inside the body, as with no **anaesthetics**, this would have been very difficult to do. One exception, however, was the draining of lungs when a patient had pneumonia. This operation was done a lot and its success was recorded for others to copy.

Source H ▼ *Greek surgical instruments. From around 1200BC, the use of iron and steel gave surgeons stronger and sharper instruments. The bleeding cup, pictured here, was used to draw blood out of a patient. The heated cup was held over a small cut and the warmth drew blood to the surface and into the cup. This treatment was used in the summer and spring when doctors thought people had too much blood in their system because they were often hot and red!*

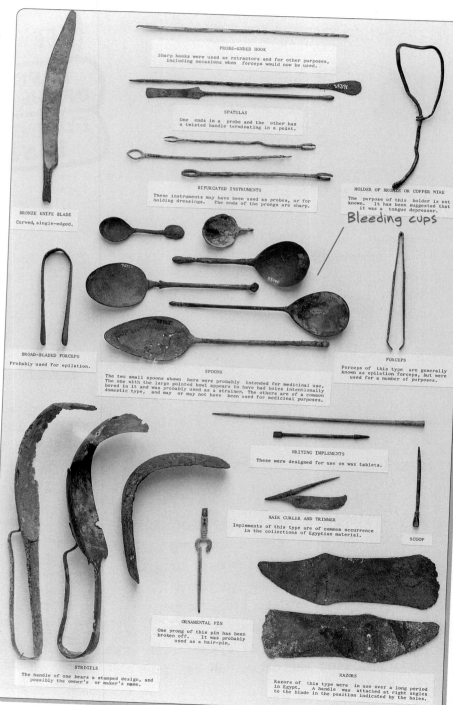

PROBE-ENDED HOOK
Sharp hooks were used as retractors and for other purposes, including occasions when forceps would now be used.

SPATULAS
One ends in a probe and the other has a twisted handle terminating in a point.

BIFURCATED INSTRUMENTS
These instruments may have been used as probes, or for holding dressings. The ends of the prongs are sharp.

HOLDER OF BRONZE OR COPPER WIRE
The purpose of this holder is not known. It has been suggested that it was a tongue depresser.

BRONZE KNIFE BLADE
Curved, single-edged.

Bleeding cups

BROAD-BLADED FORCEPS
Probably used for epilation.

SPOONS
The two small spoons shown here were probably intended for medicinal use. The one with the large pointed bowl appears to have had holes intentionally bored in it and was probably used as a strainer. The others are of a common domestic type, and may or may not have been used for medicinal purposes.

FORCEPS
Forceps of this type are generally known as epilation forceps, but were used for a number of purposes.

WRITING IMPLEMENTS
These were designed for use on wax tablets.

HAIR CURLER AND TRIMMER
Implements of this type are of common occurrence in the collections of Egyptian material.

SCOOP

ORNAMENTAL PIN
One prong of this pin has been broken off. It was probably used as a hair-pin.

STRIGILS
The handle of one bears a stamped design, and possibly the owner's or maker's name.

RAZORS
Razors of this type were in use over a long period in Egypt. A handle was attached at right angles to the blade in the position indicated by the holes.

Source I ▼ *From H Von Staden, Herophilus, the Art of Medicine in Early Alexandria, 1989.*

"The three most common 'non-magical' Egyptian techniques of wound care — putting a slab of fresh meat on a wound; applying honey and animal fat; applying adhesive linen tape — are not among the techniques used by Greeks.

The Greeks instead washed the wound with wine or vinegar — a basic **antiseptic** procedure apparently ignored in Egypt. Sometimes they bandaged wounds with linen soaked in wine."

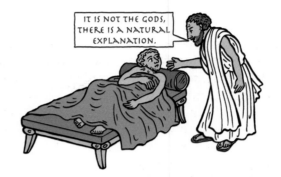

IT IS NOT THE GODS, THERE IS A NATURAL EXPLANATION.

WISE UP WORDS

- pneumonia   anaesthetics   antiseptic   dissection

FACT *What about women?*

Despite the growth in importance of doctors, women carried out most of the medical care in ancient Greece. Wives and mothers at home would use old herbal remedies handed down through the generations. This avoided the cost of going to see a doctor – which would only be done as a last resort!

FACT *Alexandria*

The Greeks conquered Egypt in the fourth century BC. The Greek leader, Alexandria the Great, built the city of Alexandria in Egypt in 331BC. A huge university and library were built there that contained medical books from India, China, Mesopotamia, Egypt and, of course, Greece. At one point, there were said to be over half a million books in the library. The university attracted medical students for hundreds of years, including Herophilus (who discovered that the brain controls the body) and Erasistratus (who discovered that the heart contained four one-way valves and worked as a kind of pump). These discoveries were made possible because **dissections** were permitted in Alexandria.

WORK

1 **a** What was new about Hippocrates' work and ideas?

   b How did Hippocrates try to spread his ideas?

   c How is his influence still felt today?

2 You have the job of training a new set of Greek doctors. Write a list – or prepare an instruction leaflet – that outlines the eight most important things they should remember. For two of your 'top tips', explain why they are so important to the success of a doctor.

3 Clearly, the ancient Greeks were developing logical explanations of disease. So why do you think healing temples and visits to a priest were still very popular in Ancient Greece?

4 Look at **Source H.** In what way did technological improvements help Greek surgeons?

5 Look at **Source I.**

   a What new treatment did the Greeks use that the Egyptians didn't?

   b Do you think this new method would have been successful or not? Explain your answer.

6 Think carefully (and this may involve looking back through your notes) – are there any theories or treatments that the Greeks practised that were:

   i) used in prehistoric times?

   ii) used in Ancient Egypt?

CLASSIC EXAM QUESTION

What breakthrough did Hippocrates make in the treatment of illness?

iii) Ancient Rome

'Here come the Romans!'

Topic Focus

▷ How Greek ideas influenced the Romans
▷ The type of treatments Roman citizens could have
▷ Roman developments in surgery.

Exam Focus

▷ How medical care was provided in early Roman history.

About 2000 years ago, the Romans conquered Greece and took over almost all of the Greek Empire. The Romans had never really thought too much about disease and medical treatment and didn't take much notice of the theories of Greek doctors such as Hippocrates. Generally speaking, they relied on simple, home-made medicines that had been used in households for generations (see **Source A**).

Source A ▾ *From* History of Medicine.

"They tried to cure diarrhoea by dosing themselves with egg yolk mixed with powdered eggshell, wine and poppy juice. This was probably quite a good treatment. The wine and the juice had a sedative (or calming) effect and the egg yolk and eggshell settled their stomachs."

Source B ▾ *The Romans 'borrowed' gods from the people they conquered, including the Greeks. When a plague swept through Rome in 295BC, they built a healing temple … dedicated to Asclepius, the Greek god of healing. A Roman official called Titus built a shrine in Chester showing Asclepius' snake winding around medical instruments. Below is an illustration of the shrine.*

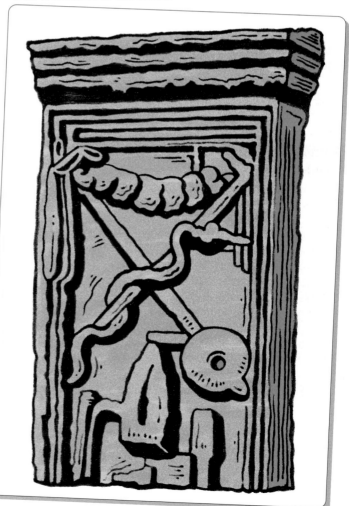

Most Romans believed that illness was caused by the gods, witchcraft and curses. Many looked for supernatural cures and travelled to healing shrines for solutions (see **Source B**). Doctors, who were almost all men and mainly Greek, were expensive … and some were total fraudsters. Anyone could call themselves a doctor, even if they'd had absolutely no medical training.

Source C ▾ *A diagram showing some of the more common medical treatments in the Roman Empire.*

Try a herbal remedy

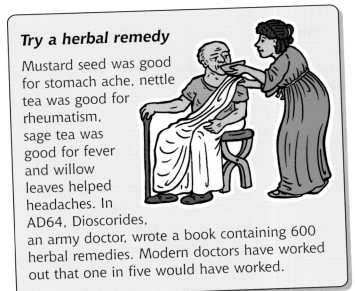

Mustard seed was good for stomach ache, nettle tea was good for rheumatism, sage tea was good for fever and willow leaves helped headaches. In AD64, Dioscorides, an army doctor, wrote a book containing 600 herbal remedies. Modern doctors have worked out that one in five would have worked.

Try the doctor

Some doctors were very well trained, spending time at the great medical libraries in Rome or Alexandria reading all about illnesses and cures. Others were con men, pretending to be doctors to make money. Travelling doctors, often old soldiers who'd done first aid in the army, visited towns to do small operations like removing a rotten tooth.

Getting better in Ancient Rome?

Offer a votive to the customer

Shops sold clay or metal models – called **votives** – of different parts of the body. You could buy a metal ear or arm (whichever part of your body hurt) and put it on the altar of the local temple and pray for a cure.

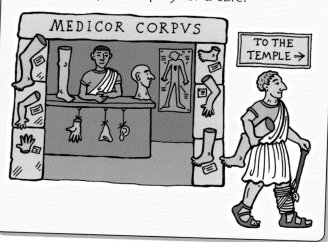

Visit the market

On market day, travelling salesmen sold bottles and jugs of medicines and healing ointments. They were often false but were sold with a promise to cure anything.

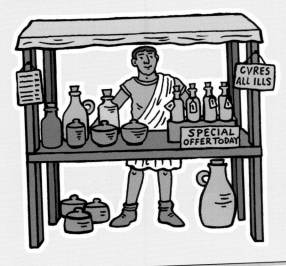

FACT *The role of women*

Women played a vital role in treating illness. As lots of treatment was done by families in their homes, the women of the house became experts on which herbs and vegetables to use to treat all sorts of ailments. There were some female doctors (one called Antiochus had a statue of herself erected in her home town!) and many successful and skilled midwives.

Source D ▾ *Pliny the Elder, a Roman writer in AD1.*

"The science of herbs is one outstanding skill of women."

Source E ▾ *The Blessing of Urine by Pliny the Elder, AD1.*

"Sores, burns, anal trouble, cracked skin and scorpion bites are also treated with urine. The greatest midwives say that no better washing material exists for skin diseases. Urine cures head wounds, dandruff and sores to the genitals. Every individual benefits most from his own urine. A dog-bite should immediately be washed with urine."

CLASSIC EXAM QUESTION

Describe how medical care was provided in the early days of Roman history.

Source F ▾ *Pliny the Elder, writing on Greek doctors in the first century AD. Romans regarded themselves as fit, strong and healthy with no need for doctors as required by the weak and feeble Greeks! Many Greek doctors were regarded as con men with fancy theories that didn't make sense. However, one Greek doctor, Asclepiades (c.120–40BC) became very popular in Rome and began to make Greek doctors respectable.*

"There is no doubt that they all risk our lives in order to be the new discoverer of some new thing to win reputations for themselves. Hence too that gloomy inscription on monuments, 'It was the crowd of doctors that killed me.' They learn by putting us in danger and make experiments until their patients die and the doctor is the only person not punished for murder."

Source G ▾ *De Medicina, book VII, a medical book compiled by Celsus in the first century AD. Despite having some quite effective drugs, Romans had no real anaesthetics. Surgery was clearly terrifying, agonising and dangerous.*

"When gangrene has developed, the limb must be amputated. But even that involves great risk; for patients often die under the operation. It does not matter however whether the remedy is safe enough, since it is the only one. Therefore, between the sound and the diseased part, the flesh is cut through with a scalpel down to the bone, but this must be done actually over a joint and it is better that some of the sound part should be cut away than any of the diseased part should be left behind ... the bone is then to be cut through with a small saw."

Source H ▾ *Some Roman medical instruments. Ow! The Romans made advances in surgery – mainly because it suited their practical needs. The Roman Empire was based on conquering land with their highly effective army so getting their injured soldiers back fighting as quickly as possible was of vital importance. One Roman writer even said that war was the best training of all for surgeons.*

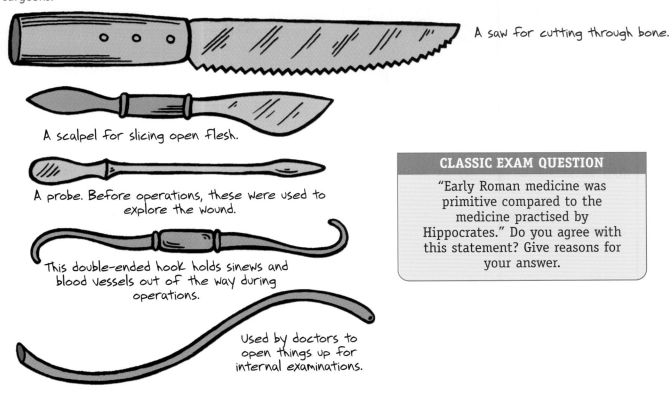

A saw for cutting through bone.

A scalpel for slicing open flesh.

A probe. Before operations, these were used to explore the wound.

This double-ended hook holds sinews and blood vessels out of the way during operations.

Used by doctors to open things up for internal examinations.

> **CLASSIC EXAM QUESTION**
>
> "Early Roman medicine was primitive compared to the medicine practised by Hippocrates." Do you agree with this statement? Give reasons for your answer.

FACT *Nothing changes!*

Celsus wrote one of the most famous books on surgery. In it, he described how to carry out plastic surgery on the nose, mouth and ears; how to clean wounds properly and how to set and treat a broken nose. Famously, he wrote down the four key signs of inflammation – redness, heat, pain and swelling – and medical students still learn this today!

FACT *Asclepiades*

One Greek doctor in particular became very popular in Rome. Asclepiades rejected Hippocrates' ideas about the four humours, claiming that the body was made up of tiny atoms always moving around the body. Between these atoms flow the body's liquids. He claimed that a person's health depended on the atoms moving smoothly and to achieve this, a person needed a balanced lifestyle – a good diet, exercise and regular bathing. Asclepiades claimed that doctors were essential to ensure that people maintained this balanced lifestyle and in time, he became one of Rome's most popular doctors.

WORK

1 **a** Which Greek god did the Romans pray to?
   b Why do you think they used some of the Greek gods?

2 Imagine your ill friend has visited you from the countryside. They want your advice on what medical treatments are available to them in Rome, the place where you live. Use **Source C** to write them a short list advising them of the sorts of treatments they might find – and the sorts of treatments they might try to avoid!

3 What roles did women play in healing the sick?

4 Read **Source G**. Do you think this patient had much chance of survival? Give reasons for your answer.

5 Why do you think Roman surgery was more advanced than Greek surgery?

Water and health

Topic Focus

▸ Understand how and why a public health system became a priority for the Romans.

Exam Focus

▸ Explain attitudes to public health in the Roman era.

Although the Romans weren't particularly interested in theories about the cause of illness, they did achieve great success in what today we would call **preventive medicine**. In other words, they did things to stop diseases from happening.

So what exactly did they do to prevent disease? What diseases were particularly common in the Roman Empire? And how did the practical skills of Roman builders produce the best public health schemes yet seen anywhere in the world?

Common sense and great skills as builders and engineers led the Romans to make a major contribution to medical development – **public health**. This means they took direct action to improve the general *health* of the *public*.

They began tackling diarrhoea and malaria, two of the most common diseases in Rome. So why were they so common? The Romans worked out that both were connected in some way with the swampy land around the city. So they set about draining the swamps and found that their health improved. They didn't really try to understand *why* the swamps were so unhealthy, they just realised that by draining them, fewer people became ill!

FACT *Killer diseases*

Today we know that diarrhoea is often caused by the germs living in dirty water (like swamp water), which contaminates drinking water or food. Malaria, an infectious disease, is caused by tiny organisms and is spread by the bites of infected mosquitoes ... that live in swamps! Romans didn't know the real cause of these diseases ... but their actions cut down the number of deaths from them!

Soon Romans realised that dirt, sewage and bad water in general were all connected with people being ill ... so decided to do something about it (see **Sources A** to **F**).

Source A ▾ *From Tony Triggs'* History of Medicine.

"When they built new cities, villages and fortresses, they avoided marshes and stagnant water, choosing instead places with plenty of fresh air and springs ... they also checked the health of local people. If they were fit and strong, the Romans felt sure that they too could live in the same area safely and drink the same water."

Source B ▾ *The Romans were sometimes forced to live in places without good water. They got round this by building huge* **aqueducts**, *like this one in Segovia, Spain, to carry water supplies into towns from sources far away in the hills.*

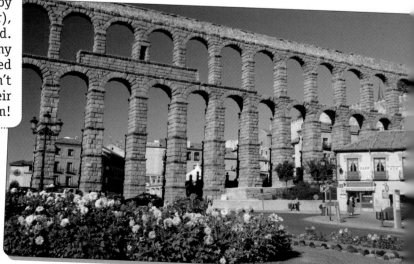

Source C ▼ *Rome itself had over 150 miles of channels taking water all over the city. This system provided 300 gallons of water a day for every person in Rome – more than each of us use today. By AD400, there were over 1000 public fountains and 144 public toilets.*

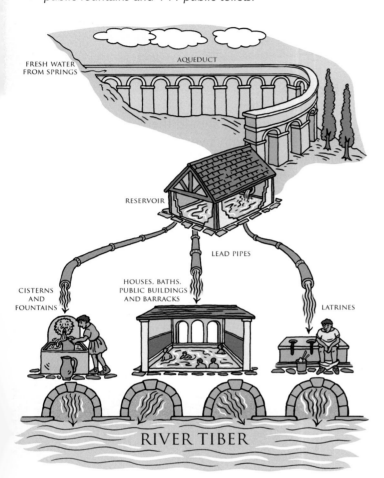

Source D ▼ *Written by Pliny, AD1.*

"If we pause to consider the huge supplies of water to public buildings, baths, pools, open channels, private houses, gardens and country estates near the city; if we think about the distance the water travels before it arrives, the raising of arches, the tunnelling of mountains, the building of level routes across valleys, we shall happily admit that there had never been anything more remarkable in the whole world."

Source E ▼ *Written by Sextus Julius Frontinus, the man in charge of water supplies in Rome in AD97. Note how he criticises the Egyptians and the Greeks.*

"As a result of the increase in the number of works, reservoirs, fountains and water basins … the air is purer and the causes of the unwholesome atmosphere, which the air of the city so bad a name … are now removed. With such an array of indispensable structures carrying so many waters, compare, if you will, the idle pyramids or the useless, though famous, works of the Greeks."

TOP EXAM TIP

The term PUBLIC HEALTH is mentioned a lot in this course. Make sure you learn what it means.

FACT *Hospitals*

The word 'hospital' comes from the Latin word *hospitalis*, meaning 'a place for guests'. The Romans didn't build many hospitals, except at forts for injured soldiers. Here they were well planned and stocked with the latest medical instruments and plenty of medical supplies.

WISE UP WORDS

• preventive medicine   public health   aqueducts

WORK

1 What is meant by the term 'preventive medicine'?
2 **a** Which illnesses were common in Rome?
  b What did the Romans do about them?
3 Imagine you work for the leaders of a large city in the ancient Roman Empire. You have been asked to design a poster explaining their public health schemes. Make sure you:
  • include a diagram
  • explain why the measures have been taken
  • summarise the effects they have had.
4 **a** What did hospitals concentrate on in Roman times?
  b Why do you think they were mostly built on the boundaries of the Roman Empire?
5 Look at **Source E**. Why did some Romans feel superior to the Greeks?

CLASSIC EXAM QUESTION

Explain attitudes to public health in Roman times.

What shall we do today?

Topic Focus

▸ After reading this double page, make sure you know how and why the Roman baths were so popular.

Most Romans agreed that people should take daily exercise to stay fit and healthy. The Roman writer Celsus wrote, 'He who has worked in the day should then take care of his body. The primary care is exercise which ought to finish with sweating!' In all Roman towns and cities, you would find public baths – a huge source of pleasure to the Romans. They were the sorts of club where rich and poor could go without paying. People went there to stay clean, treat complaints like backache, meet friends or even conduct business. You would enter the baths through the main entrance and go straight to the changing room. Then you would go to the gymnasium for some exercise. Once you had worked up a sweat, you would dive into the tepidarium (warm bath). Next, the caldarium (hot bath) where you would sweat the dirt out of your body. A slave would then rub oil over your body, massage out any aches and pains, then scrape away the dirt with a strigil (a metal scraper). You would then pop back into the tepidarium and then into the frigidarium (cold bath). You might then go into the natatio (swimming pool) for a swim before enjoying a glass of wine with friends in one of the bars.

In some of the bigger cities, the baths might also contain shops, a racetrack, circus, theatre and even a gladiator arena! Baths were so popular that they were often the first public building put up in a new town.

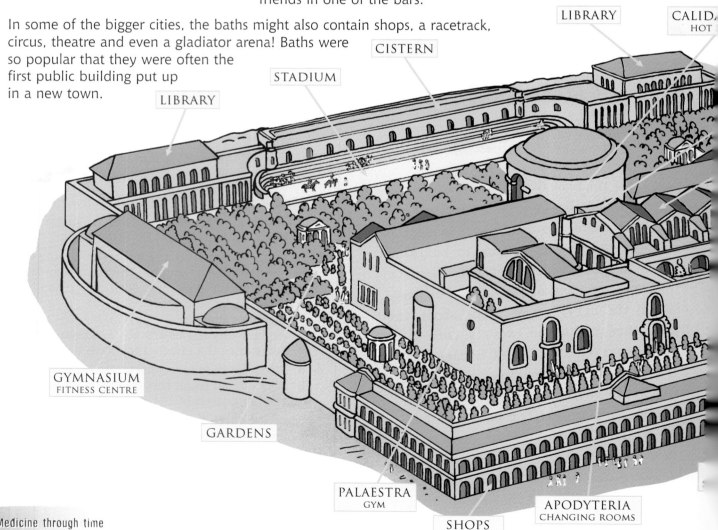

LIBRARY

CALID/
HOT

CISTERN

STADIUM

LIBRARY

GYMNASIUM
FITNESS CENTRE

GARDENS

PALAESTRA
GYM

SHOPS

APODYTERIA
CHANGING ROOMS

Source B ▾ *Seneca, a Roman writer, who lived near the public baths.*

" Just imagine every kind of annoying noise. The fat, old gentleman does his workout with lead weights. When he's working hard, or pretending to, I can hear him grunting; when he's out of breath, I can hear him panting. Or I might notice some idle dog, happy to have a cheap rub down and hear the blows of the hands slapping his shoulders … to all this you can add the noise of the man singing in his bath and the chap who leaps in with a hell of a lot of shouting and splashing! On top of this, the hair-plucker shouts out too loudly to catch our attention. "

FACT *What about Britain?*

When the Romans invaded Britain, they brought their aqueducts, public baths, racetracks, theatres and arenas with them. Towns like Wroxeter were supplied by aqueducts, stone sewers were built in York and Bath had a … bath!

FACT *Not perfect though!*

Roman public health was impressive – but not perfect. Many poor Romans lived in crowded areas where disease spread easily. In the second century AD, there was a smallpox outbreak that killed over 2000 people a day at its height. And Rome's famous sewers emptied into the river Tiber … which must have been horrible for people further up the river who relied on the water to cook and wash their clothes!

WORK

1 **a** In your own words, describe Roman public baths in the days of the Empire.

b Why do you think that the public baths were usually one of the first buildings to be built in new towns?

c How do Roman public baths differ from the swimming baths we are used to today?

2 Look at **Source B**. In your opinion, do you think the writer of the source likes living near the public baths or not? Give reasons for your answer, using quotes from the source where appropriate.

3 The Romans believed in preventive medicine. Do public baths fit in with this theory? Give reasons for your answer.

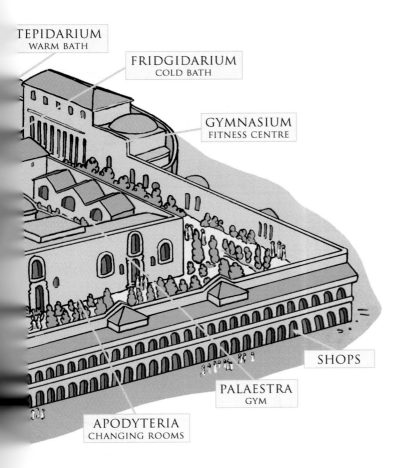

TEPIDARIUM WARM BATH
FRIDGIDARIUM COLD BATH
GYMNASIUM FITNESS CENTRE
SHOPS
PALAESTRA GYM
APODYTERIA CHANGING ROOMS

◄ **Source A** *The baths of Caracalla in Rome covered 33 acres (about 18 football pitches) and had a stadium as well as room for 1600 bathers at a time.*

Galen the Great?

Topic Focus

> Do you know why Galen is so important in medical history, and did he get anything wrong?

Exam Focus

> What developments in medicine were made by Galen?

In AD162, a Greek doctor travelled to Rome in search of fame and fortune. He was known as Galen. At 33 years old, he had been studying medicine for over 15 years. He had gained masses of practical experience in treating all sorts of vicious wounds when serving as a surgeon at a gladiators' school. He knew how to treat gaping cuts, smashed bones and severed fingers. He had also developed some interesting theories about health and medicine … and now he wanted to make a name for himself (and make some money too!). His first move was typically bold and soon got the whole of Rome talking about him (see **Source A**).

Source A ▾

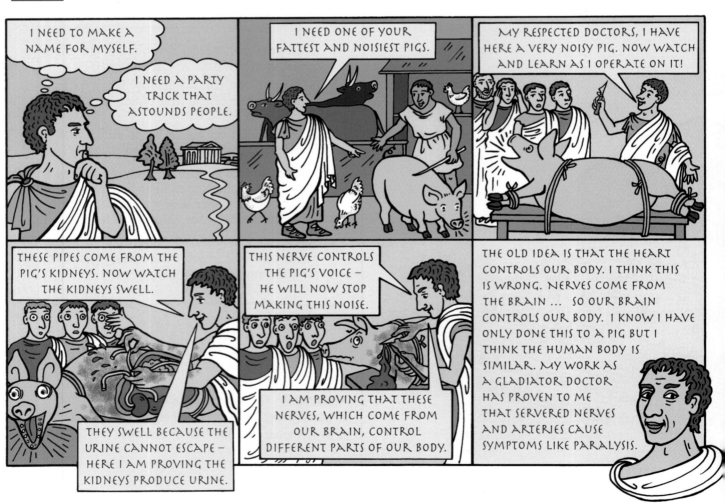

Galen's experiments worked for him. They made him the talk of Rome and he became the city's most famous doctor. He especially impressed the Romans by treating people that other doctors couldn't cure (see **Source B**). Within a year, he had become the Emperor's doctor … and remained in the royal household for the rest of his life.

Source B ▾ *Tony Triggs'* History of Medicine.

"A Persian philosopher, who lived in Rome, was suffering from numbness in three of his fingers. Other doctors had given him ointments but Galen asked him if he had had any injuries. The Persian replied that he had hit the upper part of his back on a sharp piece of rock. Galen said that he must have damaged his spine in the place where the finger nerves branch off. He told the man to rest in bed and apply his ointment to his back. Sure enough, the feeling soon came back to his fingers."

Galen's ideas and methods

Patients flocked to Galen for treatment. He rescued the ideas and methods of Hippocrates (which the Romans hadn't really taken any notice of) and told doctors to observe, record and use their experience of past cases to work out how to treat their patients. He was well known for spending hours talking to patients about their lifestyle … before examining their blood, urine and even their poo!

Galen also believed in the theory of the four humours and that any treatment should aim to restore the balance of these humours.

He recommended 'opposites' to restore balance in a patient's body. For example, if a patient had a cold and had lots of phlegm running down their nose, Galen would tell them to take pepper. Why? Because phlegm is cold and wet so the 'opposite' treatment should be hot and fiery … so pepper was ideal!

Galen's books

Galen wrote over 350 books. He even employed 20 people to write down everything he said. Much of it was a summary of what Hippocrates had said years before but he presented it so well that no one really questioned his ideas or treatment for the next 1500 years.

Galen's influence

Galen's careful dissections of pigs, dogs and apes meant he discovered lots of new information about **anatomy**. He dissected some humans but usually had to make do with animals. As a result, he had to base his theories about us on his animal experiments … which meant he made mistakes. For example, he claimed that the human jaw is made from two separate bones – correct for an animal but wrong for a human. Our jaws are made from a single bone! However, Galen's books do show a very good understanding of anatomy but a limited understanding of physiology (the way various organs work). One of Galen's most famous mistakes was to think the heart was divided into two parts, each carrying two separate lots of blood around the body. He also believed that the liver made new blood from food. People believed Galen's wrong ideas for the next 1500 years. By claiming to be the greatest expert on the human body ever, medical progress was prevented as his mistakes were passed on … and many doctors stopped researching into new theories. After all, what was the point if Galen had already found all the answers?

FACT *Time of the month!*

Galen was famous for encouraging bloodletting as a treatment for almost any disease. Many complaints, from fever to bad temperedness, were put down to having too much blood in the body … which needed a serious bleeding session to sort things out. He even said that women were protected from many diseases because they menstruated!

TOP EXAM TIP

Make sure you understand Galen's importance, both in his own lifetime and also how he affected medicine in the future.

FACT *The Church*

The Christian Church taught that Galen's work was correct. Galen felt that every natural thing had a definite purpose so this appealed to Christian leaders who felt that God was an almighty designer. So if the Church approved Galen's work, no one was likely to challenge it! Galen himself wasn't a Christian or a Muslim but believed in one God and talked of a 'creator'. This made his work acceptable to Islamic cultures too.

Source C ▼ *The title page of one of Galen's books, published in 1565.*

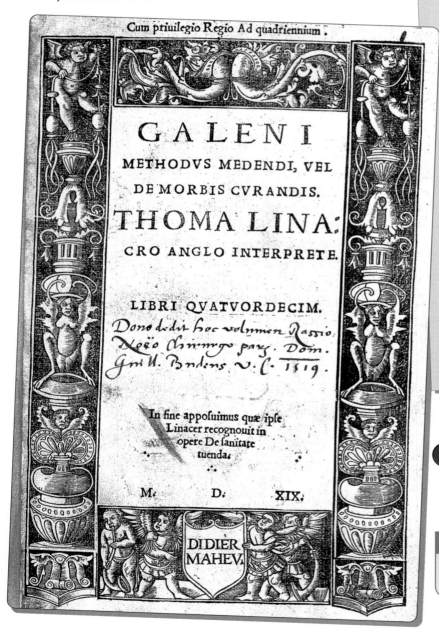

Source D ▼ *From a book by Galen called* On Anatomy, *AD190.*

"Human bones are subjects of study with which you should become familiar. And don't just read about bones in books — even in my book, which is far more reliable than any previous books!

At Alexandria, this is very easy since the doctors let their students watch them at post-mortems. But if you cannot get to Alexandria, it is still possible to study human bones. I have often done this when tombs of the dead have been broken into and I once examined the skeleton of a dead robber left lying by the side of the road. If you don't have any luck seeing anything like this, then cut up an ape instead. And choose apes that resemble men."

WISE UP WORD

- anatomy

CLASSIC EXAM QUESTION

What knowledge of anatomy and surgery was there in Ancient Rome?

Source E ▼ *Galen, writing about himself in a typically 'big-headed' way.*

"I have done as much for medicine as Trojan did for the Roman Empire when he built bridges and roads through Italy. It is I, and I alone, who have revealed the true methods of treating disease. It must be admitted that Hippocrates prepared the way, but he did not follow it up; his works have grave limitations. He marked out the road; I have made it passable."

SUMMARY

- The Ancient Egyptians, Greeks and Romans thought gods caused disease. Greeks and Romans believed in the theory of the four humours.

- They all performed simple surgery and used herbal remedies. All emphasised the importance of personal hygiene but the Romans carried on large public health programmes.

- Priests, doctors and family members (especially women) treated the sick.

- Key individuals, like Hippocrates and Galen, developed their theories during this period.

CLASSIC EXAM QUESTION

The Greeks and Romans were equally interested in discovering the causes of disease." Explain why you agree or disagree with this statement.

WORK

1 **a** What work did Galen do at gladiator school?
   b What did it teach him?

2 Look at **Source A**.
   a What did Galen do:
      i) to the pipes that led from a pig's kidneys?
      ii) to the nerves that control the pig's voice?
      In each case, explain what Galen noticed and why it occurred.
   b Why do you think Galen decided to operate on a noisy pig and invite lots of doctors?

3 Look at **Source B**. Explain why some doctors told the patient to put ointment on his fingers but Galen told him to put it on his back.

4 **a** Galen was wrong about a number of things. Give two examples.
   b Why do you think he was wrong about these things?

5 Read the fact box entitled 'The Church'. How did religion hinder medical progress?

6 Read **Source D**.
   a What basic advice does it give the readers of this book?
   b How did Galen himself get experience of working with human bones when he was younger?
   c Is there anything in this passage that backs up the theory that Galen was a 'big-headed' doctor?

7 Copy out and complete the following chart, which compares Greek and Roman ideas about medicine. You may have to look back over all your notes on Roman medicine to complete it properly. The first one has been done for you.

Greek medicine	Did the Romans use this idea or method?	Example
The gods could cure illness and disease	Romans agreed that gods could cure illness and disease	They prayed to the gods, sometimes building shrines and temples. They even 'borrowed' the Greek god Asclepius.
Herbal medicines were commonly used		
Doctors talked to their patients, examined them and recorded their findings		
Good diet, exercise and regular bathing were encouraged		
Doctors worked hard to discover the cause of disease		
Doctors could perform basic operations		

Studying Sources Made Simple

Many of your history lessons over the years will have featured **SOURCES** in some way. Quite simply a source is a piece of information. A source can be a document, a painting, a photograph, poster, chart, diary entry, speech, even a group of statistics ... in fact anything that provides us with information. In your exam you will almost certainly be asked questions about any number of sources that appear on the exam paper in front of you. The sources might be charts used by medieval doctors, diagrams from ancient medical books, speeches by famous surgeons, quotes from old textbooks or copies of doctors' notes from the twentieth century.

There are five main types of source question – and your first job when confronted with a source question is to work out what type of question it is!

Source question type 1: Extraction

An EXTRACTION question challenges the student to get as much out of the source as they can.

Typical questions:

- What can we learn from Sources A and B about ... ?
- What does Source D tell us about... ?

Top tips

- Make sure you understand the source – read it slowly and carefully, including the label (or provenance, as it is sometimes known)
- Write down what the source tells us about the specific issue asked in the question. For example, if you are asked what a source tells us about the way doctors found out about illness – make sure you write down at least three things that the source tells you
- Try to write down what you can infer from the source. For example, is there a message in the source? Is it trying to create an impression by trying to make you think in a certain way?
- Also, what does the source tell you about the author, the time it was written and/or the situation in which it was written?

Source question type 2: Similarities and differences

A SIMILARITY/DIFFERENCE question asks a student to compare and contrast a number of sources

Typical questions:

- Do the sources agree about... ?
- In what way do Sources A and B differ about... ?
- Why is Source A's interpretation different to Source B's?

Top tips

- If asked HOW two sources are similar or different, look for basic things to compare – mention what they agree on for example, and what they disagree on! Also look for differences and/or similarities in tone, approach, message etc.
- If asked WHY the sources are similar or different, you need to look carefully at the label that accompanies the source. Look who wrote it, and when, and in what context or situation. Think why it was written and for what purpose.
- Wherever possible here, use quotes from the sources to back up the point you are trying to make ... and write a conclusion to your answer too, summing up how and/or why they are similar or different.

Source question type 3: Reliability

RELIABILITY questions want students to judge how accurate and reliable a source is.

Typical questions:

- How accurate is Source C as a source of information... ?
- How reliable is... ?

Top tips

- Try to establish the extent to which the source might be biased or exaggerated. Look at the words, phrases and language. Use your own knowledge here – does the source give you an accurate picture of things? Compare it to other sources that might be available.
- Look at the label to establish who wrote it and when. Try to judge how one sided or exaggerated it might be. Think whether it gives the whole story and point out, from your own knowledge, what it misses out! Is the writer trying to 'make a point' for example? Do they have a reason or motive to lie?
- Make sure you come to a conclusion here, based on facts. And try to avoid general phrases like 'it is biased' without backing it up with evidence. For example write 'it would be biased because ...' instead.

Source question type 5: Final conclusions

Exam papers often include CONCLUSION questions which ask students to use all the sources. The question often asks students to debate a particular issue, or proposition, and use the sources to back up their conclusion.

Typical questions:

- Use all the sources to debate...
- Do all the sources agree that public health improved at different times for different reasons?

Top tips

- Look through all the sources again with the question in mind.
- The sources have been selected to support both sides of the argument, or position, use them to argue both for and against, making sure you take into account the accuracy and reliability of the sources you use to reach your conclusion.

Source question type 4: Utility

UTILITY questions ask how useful a source is. 'Utility' is just another way of asking how 'useful' a source is to a historian studying that particular period of time.

Typical question:

- How useful is Source D to an Historian studying surgery in the Middle Ages?

Top tips

- Utility questions are all about QUANTITY and QUALITY – how much information does it give you, and how reliable is that information? The most reliable source, therefore, is one that tells you a lot and you can trust what it says!
- Think about what the source tells you ... and think whether it's actually the sort of information you're looking for in relation to the question.
- Look at the sufficiency of the source – does it give you the whole story? Explain the source's limitations – as well as explaining what it is used for.
- Think about who produced it, why, and whether you can trust them. If you can trust a source – you must explain why! And just because a source is widely inaccurate in what it says, doesn't mean it isn't useful – it perhaps reveals a lot about the author's feelings, prejudices and opinions. In fact, nothing is ever useless, no matter how biased it is. Remember that the source reveals lots about the individual or the government of the organisation that produces it.

FACT *Think SOURCE when evaluating one*

Source – Where is it from? When was it written? Who is the author?

Objective –Why was it written? For a diary, a newspaper, a speech?

Usefulness – What use is it for the question you are answering?

Reliability – Can you trust it? If so why/why not?

Context – What was going on at the time it was written? Put the source into context. Use your background knowledge here.

Example – Always use an example from the source to back up what you have written.

Getting better after the Romans?

Topic Focus

This topic looks at:
> Whether there was any improvement in health and medicine in the Middle Ages
> What happened to the ideas the Greeks and Romans had about medicine.

Exam Focus

> Understand what people in Anglo Saxon times understood about the cause and cure of illness.

The Romans invaded the British Isles in AD43. They quickly captured the southern parts of England but struggled to conquer the north and Wales where the countryside was hilly and where tribesmen could hide in the dense forests. Instead, they just built dozens of forts in an attempt to keep order and stationed most of their army where the most rebellious tribes lived. The people of Scotland, known as Pits, were never conquered.

The Romans remained in Britain for almost 400 years and, generally speaking, Britain became a more peaceful place as fighting between different tribes was stopped, quarrels were settled in court and people travelled around quicker and in safety.

When the Romans left in about AD400, tribes from northern Europe called Angles, Saxons and Jutes invaded. Some people called the years after the Romans 'the Dark Ages' because it was when there was a lot of fighting and destruction. The new invaders fought and beat some of the fiercer tribes still around in Britain, eventually making some of them slaves. Other British tribes made peace with the new invaders and settled down to live side by side. Although there seems to have been more invading Saxon tribesmen than Angles or Jutes, the country we now call England gradually became known as Angleland – and the people who lived there were called Anglo-Saxons.

So how healthy were the Anglo-Saxons? Did medicine grow worse after the Romans? In fact, how 'dark' were the Dark Ages in terms of health and medicine?

Life was tough in Anglo-Saxon times – very tough. In a cemetery in Kent, dating from about AD600, archaeologists recently found 32 skeletons. Experts worked out that 23 of the people had died before they were 30; eight between 30 and 45; and only one was over 45. Today, the average age of death is over 75. So, why did the Anglo-Saxons die so young? (Read **Sources A** and **B** to find out.)

Source A ▾

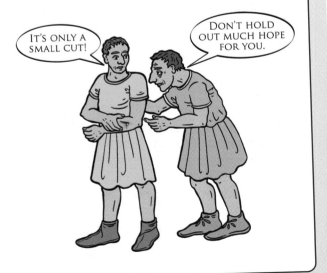

Terrible treatment

In Roman times, the largest towns were filled with medical books giving details about diet and fitness, herbal treatments and instructions on diagnosing and curing illness. But the tribes who followed them couldn't read them so there was no real medical treatment except herbs. People would have died of infections from small cuts and minor illnesses.

IT'S ONLY A SMALL CUT!

DON'T HOLD OUT MUCH HOPE FOR YOU.

Dodgy diet

Each family grew its own food and there were no shops if they ran out! They mainly ate bread, beans, peas, barley and wheat — not a bad diet but lacking in red meat. As a result, they lacked crucial vitamins … which lowered their resistance to disease.

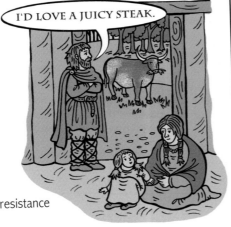

I'D LOVE A JUICY STEAK.

Horrible housing

Most families lived in a dark, damp, one-room draughty hut. The animals lived in the hut too! There was no running water and the toilet was a hole in the ground outside. Diseases like dysentery (an infection that causes severe diarrhoea … and can kill) were common.

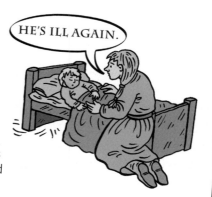

HE'S ILL AGAIN.

Rotten work

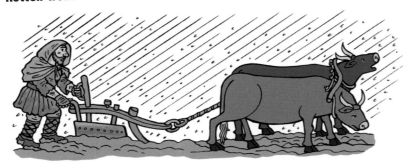

They worked in all weathers, all day, all year round — clearing forests, ploughing land, sowing seeds, harvesting crops and so on. Their one set of clothes could stay wet through for weeks on end. Cuts would get dirty and infected and severe joint pain (arthritis and rheumatism) was common.

TOP EXAM TIP

Make sure you can work out how each of these key factors might affect health.

Furious fighting

There was always danger — fights against robbers, wild animals or even other kingdoms. Fighting was brutal too — with no real medical treatment for even the smallest wounds.

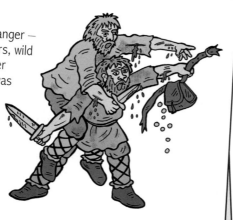

Pesky plague

Animal plagues often killed their stock. This would mean less food and less clothing. And if the prospect of their animals dying wasn't bad enough, if the animals were alive then their owners could catch diseases from them — skin infections for example.

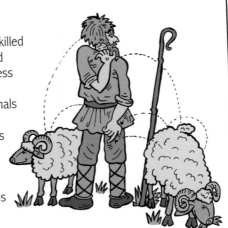

But we mustn't think that the Anglo-Saxons were stupid because they couldn't read Roman and Greek books or didn't work out that unhealthy living conditions and dirt were linked to poor health. Anglo-Saxon doctors had the same problems as Roman and Greek doctors – there were no effective painkillers (although herbs like mandrake and poppy would have dulled some of the pain) and no really useful antiseptics. As a result, many people would have suffered in agony from ailments like toothache or cracked bones and many even died from small wounds that became badly infected.

Yet Anglo-Saxon healers *did* use some effective treatments made from plants and minerals ... they knew the treatments worked, but just didn't know how! For example:

- onions and garlic were rubbed into cuts that hurt (we know today that these kill some bacteria);
- willow leaves were used to treat headaches (we know today that the leaves contain a painkiller similar to aspirin).

Source C – *From a modern history book.*

"Although the Anglo-Saxons had no idea what was causing disease, many of the medicines they used were natural treatments and did help patients to recover. Some of these were copied from the Romans and some they developed themselves through long and careful observation ... treatments like these were effective and it was no accident that the Anglo-Saxon doctors used them."

She was 157cm or 5 feet 2 inches tall.

Most of her teeth had rotted away leaving just the roots. There were no dentists to visit or toothpaste and mouthwash to use. Eating must have been agony for her.

A broken collarbone was identified. It had healed well which shows that Anglo-Saxons probably knew how to set broken bones properly.

She would have had back pain. Her skeleton shows signs of arthritis. This would have made everyday jobs very difficult.

By analysing the pelvis, experts can tell she was female. She was actually born with a deformed pelvis.

By measuring the length of some of her bones, experts can tell she died in her 30s.

Source B ▸ *An Anglo-Saxon skeleton. Interestingly, most skeletons dated to Roman times (hundreds of years before Anglo-Saxon times) and found in heavily populated Roman areas like York, show <u>no</u> signs of diseases caused by poor diets. They were well supplied with meat and bread, as well as imported goods like grapes and olives from the Empire. However, many of the skeletons were young – showing it was impossible to protect babies and children from many of the most common infectious diseases.*

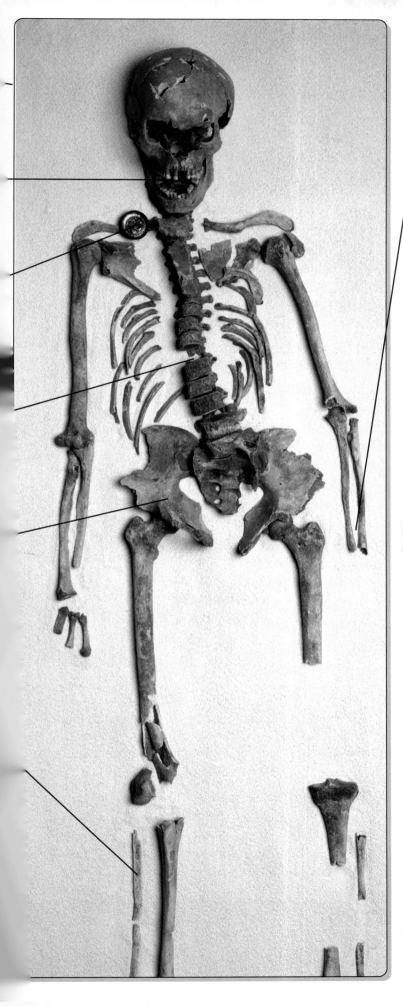

She wore a bronze bracelet on her wrist. Magic was an important part of Anglo-Saxon medicine and was used alongside natural, herbal remedies. People would have routinely worn special bracelets, necklaces and amulets (a charm that the wearer thinks will give them protection against disease).

Source D ▾ *A modern historian, writing about the Anglo-Saxons.*

"A fairly short life expectancy, a high infant mortality, women dying young, particularly in childbirth and a fairly high incidence of bone and joint diseases such as rheumatism, arthritis and rickets."

WORK

1 **a** How do you think 'the Dark Ages' gets its name?

  b Who were the Anglo-Saxons?

2 Why are bones an excellent source to study for historians interested in health and medicine long ago?

3 Look at **Source B**. Imagine you are one of a team of archaeologists who helped to dig up the remains of the woman pictured in **Source B**. Write an archaeologist's report about the woman, describing in detail the injuries she sustained during her lifetime and an explanation of how her lifestyle may have led to these injures. Conclude with your general theories as to why she (and many like her) died so young. You will need to use the cartoons and text on pages 40 and 41 to help you complete this task properly.

CLASSIC EXAM QUESTION

What did people in Anglo-Saxon times understand about the cause and cure of illness?

Medicine in the Muslim world

Topic Focus

> To understand the quality and extent of Islamic medical knowledge.

Exam Focus

> To be able to compare and contrast Arab medicine with European medicine at this time.

As the Roman Empire declined and fierce tribes fought each other all over Europe (a time known as the Dark Ages), a new civilisation was growing in the Middle East. Based on the Islamic faith, Arab Muslims took a special interest in medicine. In fact, the Koran, the holiest Islamic book containing the words of Mohammed, tells Arab Muslims to take good care of the sick and those in need.

So what did Muslims know about health and medicine? How did they gain their knowledge and understanding? And was Islamic medicine more advanced than European medicine?

How did they gain their knowledge?

Arab Muslims learned from the people they conquered and the books they kept. Caliph al-Ma'mun (ruled AD813–833) built a House of Wisdom – a sort of university – in Baghdad and his workers translated medical books written by ancient Greeks and Romans like Hippocrates and Galen. The books contained ideas more advanced than Islamic medicine at the time and Muslims were happy to learn from them. They also searched for books as far away as Africa and India – and many of these books would have been lost forever if the Muslims hadn't translated them into Arabic.

Who were the famous Muslim doctors and surgeons?

* **Rhazes** (born in Persia in AD865)

   He agreed with Hippocrates and Galen who stressed the need to carefully observe the patient, study the disease and base any treatment on what you see. However, he did warn against the dangers of blindly following the works of Hippocrates and Galen when he wrote, "What is written in books is not worth as much as the experience of a wise doctor." Rhazes himself wrote over 100 books on medicine (see **Source A**).

Source A ▾ Rhazes, On Smallpox and Measles, c.AD900. This extract clearly illustrates how important Rhazes thought observation was. In fact, this is one of the first ever recorded observations of these two illnesses.

> "The outbreak of smallpox is preceded by continuous fever, aching in the back and shivering during sleep. The main symptoms are backache, fever, stinging pains, violent redness of the cheeks and eyes and a difficulty breathing and coughing. Excitement, nausea and unrest are more pronounced in measles than in smallpox, while the aching of the back is more severe."

* **Ibn Sina** (born in Persia in AD980)

   Known as Avicenna in Europe, he wrote a million-word book on medicine. It contained all sorts of treatments for all known diseases and was used by trainee doctors as a textbook until the 1600s!

* **Abulcasis** (born in Spain in AD936)

   Translated ideas of Paul of Aegina, a Greek medical writer who described how to do simple surgery. Soon, Muslim surgeons improved on his methods (see **Source B**).

TOP EXAM TIP

The examiner will want to see how much you know about the quality of Western European medical knowledge compared to that of the Islamic Empire: you must be confident you know this.

Source B ▾ *From Understanding History.*

"They could operate on veins and remove cancers. They used tubes as stomach drains to remove fluids and they could amputate arms and legs when necessary. They used anaesthetics, like opium, and operated on eyes to remove cataracts. Eye diseases are common in the Middle East and this became a special skill of Muslim doctors."

Source C ▾ *This story was written down by a wealthy Muslim called Usamah ibn Munqidh who lived from 1095 to 1188, the time of the Crusades. Muslims and Europeans had direct contact with each other during this time and this story shows the stark contrast between the two cultures. Over time however, many new important Muslim ideas came into Europe as people returned from the Crusades.*

"An Arab doctor was asked to treat a knight with a cut on his leg and a woman with lung disease. He cleaned the knight's leg and put a fresh dressing on it and changed the woman's diet to make her feel better.

A European doctor appeared and laughed at the Arab doctor's ideas. He told the knight that it would be better for him to live with one leg than not to live at all and ordered that the wounded leg should be removed. The knight died with one swing of the axe.

The European doctor then cut open the woman's skull and removed her brain. He rubbed the brain with salt, claiming that this would wash away the devil inside her. The woman, of course, died instantly."

Did they have hospitals?

As stated, part of the Muslim faith is to care for the sick and those in need. As a result, there were over 30 large hospitals built in Baghdad, Cairo and other cities. They contained separate wards for different illnesses and 'out patients' departments for people who didn't need to stay in hospital. Most doctors treated the poor without charge but earned huge sums from their wealthy patients. Travelling clinics toured the areas outside large towns and from AD931, doctors in Baghdad had to pass an exam to get a licence.

How were patients treated?

Doctors worked on their patients in a variety of ways. Some looked at astrological charts and recommended prayer to heal the sick. More common though was thorough examination – checking urine, their pulse and lifestyle. They used a variety of drugs made from animal and plant extracts and from chemicals like copper sulphate (we know today that this makes an excellent ointment for infected eyelids!). In some cities, inspectors checked the quality of the drugs – and a chemist caught cheating his customer could be beaten!

Source D ▸ *A picture from a book by al-Biruni, an Arab Muslim scientist. Dated around 1300, it is the earliest known picture of a baby being born by Caesarean section.*

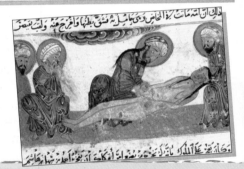

WORK

1   How did Arab Muslims learn about health and medicine?

2   Write a brief note about why you think each of the following was important: i) Caliph al-Ma'mun ii) Rhazes   iii) Avicenna   iv) Abulcasis

3   Look at **Source C**.

   a   In your own words, describe why both the patients died, despite the attention of two doctors.

   b   Who appears to have the best understanding of medicine – the European doctor or the Arab doctor? Explain your answer.

   c   Why do you think medical knowledge in Europe might have improved after many years of fighting against Muslims in the Crusades?

4   Are there any similarities between the way Arab and European doctors treated their patients?

CLASSIC EXAM QUESTION

Compare and contrast Arab medicine with European medicine at this time.

Welcome to London

Topic Focus
▸ Be able to describe the state of public health in a typical medieval town.

Exam Focus
▸ How were Roman towns healthier than medieval ones?

Today, there are lots of regulations linked to health and hygiene. Laws cover all sorts of things like sewage disposal, rubbish collection and water supplies. In the Middle Ages, however, there were very few regulations and they were very hard to enforce (no police force you see!).

And the quality of food was pretty bad too. There was no such thing as a refrigerator and butchers kept their meat on show on their market stalls. In warm weather, the smell of rotting meat must have been terrible … and flies must have been attracted to it from miles around.

Look carefully at this picture of a typical London street scene in the Middle Ages.

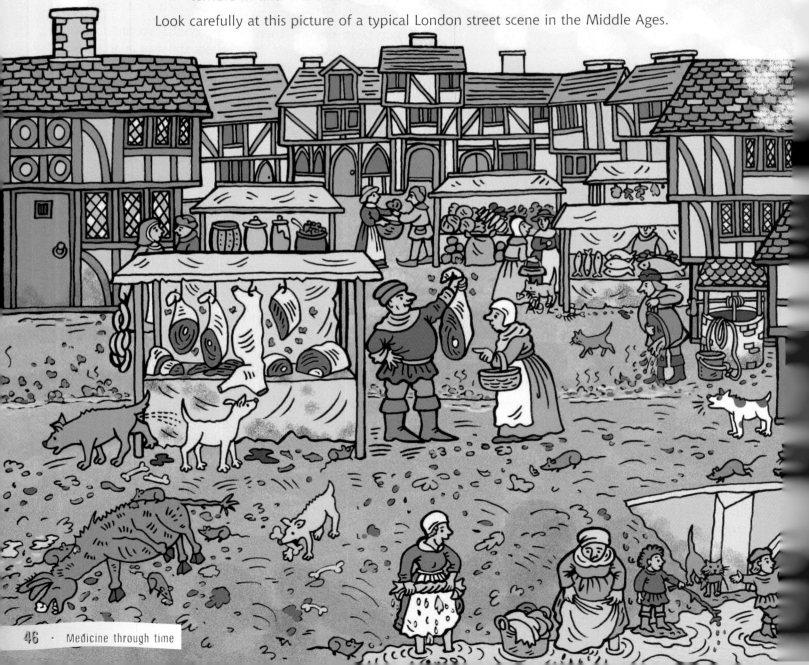

Source A ▼ *Even King Edward III was disgusted with London. This is part of a letter he wrote to the Mayor. The letter is important to historians because it shows that people at the time were beginning to make a link between dirt and disease! Yes, they thought it was the 'bad air' that caused disease, not germs, but at least a link had been established.*

"...the streets and lanes through which people had to pass were foul with human **faeces** and the air of the city poisoned to the great danger of men passing."

WISE UP WORD

- faeces

CLASSIC EXAM QUESTION

a Describe the state of public health in medieval towns.

b How were Roman towns healthier than medieval towns?

Some attempts were made to make the city a cleaner place. In 1372, anyone who had filth outside their house could be fined four shillings and there was a ban on throwing anything out of a window. Teams of 'gong farmers' were employed to collect dung (or 'gong') from the streets ... and then sell it to farmers! Even tradesmen were targeted – a London by-law stated that butchers were not allowed to sell meat that was 'putrid, rotten and stinking.'

WORK

1 Make a list of at least eight dangers to health in the picture. For each one, explain how it is unhygienic or a danger to the health of London's citizens.

2 **a** In what ways did the government in London at least try to make the city healthier?

   b Why do you think they made these efforts?

3 **a** What is meant by the word 'regress'?

   b Explain how changes in public health between the Ancient World (particularly the Romans) and the Middle Ages show 'regress'.

Trust me, I'm a doctor!

Topic Focus

▸ Understand the types of health care available in the Middle Ages.

Exam Focus

▸ Be able to describe how a medieval doctor might diagnose and treat illness.

It is 1350 and you feel ill. You go to the doctor – but he has no modern drugs or medicine to give you and doesn't know that germs and viruses cause disease. In fact, he doesn't know much about the real cause of illness at all.

So what will he do to make you feel better?

To find out what is wrong with you, he would probably ask you to urinate in a bottle. He will examine it three times: once when it is fresh, again when it has been cooled for about an hour and, lastly, when it has gone completely cold. He might even taste it to see if it was sweet or sour, bitter or salty. He would probably examine your blood, look at your tongue and take your pulse. He might even ask you to poo on a tray so he could have a good look through it!

Your doctor would then go off to consult his charts. The colour of your urine would be checked against the shades on a special diagram. They did this because they wrongly thought that every shade had a definite meaning.

Source A ▾ Urine charts and books.

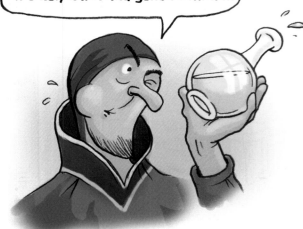

It's wet, warm and yellow I think...

FACT *Surgery*

Surgeons were often viewed as no better than butchers. They didn't need to go to university but did need to pass a test to get their licence. They pulled teeth, lanced boils, treated burns, set broken bones and let blood. Military surgeons were experts at removing arrowheads and repairing cuts.

Your doctor would believe that your illness could be explained with the ancient 'theory of the four humours' – that your body contains four substances called humours: blood, phlegm, black bile and yellow bile. When all four are present in equal amounts, the body is healthy. When they are out of balance, you become ill. Age, diet, lifestyle and even the weather could all upset this balance. It would be your doctor's task to put the balance right. Too little of a humour meant it must be topped up; too much meant some must be let out. And everything was explained by this theory – a red swelling meant too much blood, a runny nose meant too much phlegm and a hard dark lump meant too much black bile (and to this day, no one really knows what black bile was!). Each humour had certain characteristics – blood was hot and wet, phlegm was cold and wet, black bile was cold and dry, yellow bile was hot and dry. As a result, any medicine you were given was designed to get the humours back into balance. Medicine was divided into four types:

- warming
- cooling
- moistening
- drying (see **Source B**).

Source B ▾ *Humours and solutions.*

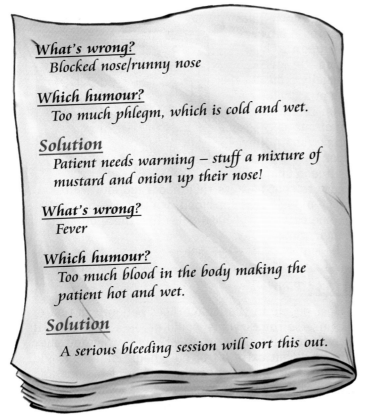

What's wrong?
Blocked nose/runny nose

Which humour?
Too much phlegm, which is cold and wet.

Solution
Patient needs warming – stuff a mixture of mustard and onion up their nose!

What's wrong?
Fever

Which humour?
Too much blood in the body making the patient hot and wet.

Solution
A serious bleeding session will sort this out.

Your doctor would have access to all sorts of strange mixtures and potions. He would look them up in his medical books or delve into his notes for any old traditional recipes. You might be given a mixture of plants, animals or minerals to swallow, or ointments made from wax or grease to rub into affected areas. Plants like clover, poppy, willow leaves and garlic were used a lot. So was honey and wine. Sugar, ginger and nutmeg were imported from places like India and Egypt.

Source C ▾ *Some strange mixtures and potions must have left their patients wondering how they related to the four humours and how on earth they would put them back into balance! Check out these genuine 'cures' from the Middle Ages.*

Toothache – burn a candle near the tooth. Hold a bowl of cold water underneath to catch the tooth-eating worms.

Warts – hold a live toad next to the skin to soften it.

Boils – cut a pigeon in half and rub it into the swollen area.

Coughing – drink the blood of a black cat; mix it with milk.

Fainting – burn feathers and breathe in the smoke.

Source D ▾ *Specialist medicine makers – called* **apothecaries** *– were incredibly successful. Today, we know that their use of herbs and plants must have had real success. Modern scientists have analysed a leechbook (a medical book from Anglo-Saxon times) and concluded that over half the herbal remedies prescribed to ease pain and help fight infection would have actually worked!*

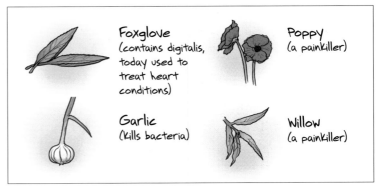

Foxglove (contains digitalis, today used to treat heart conditions)
Poppy (a painkiller)
Garlic (kills bacteria)
Willow (a painkiller)

CLASSIC EXAM QUESTION
Explain how doctors in the Middle Ages might find out about a patient's health.

If you were particularly unlucky, your doctor might insist on **purging** you to get rid of unwanted humours. He might give you something to make you vomit or even give you an enema (a mixture of water, wheat bran, salt, honey and soap) that was squirted up your bottom through a greasy pipe!

Source E ⮟ *A patient made to 'vomit' by his doctor to get rid of an excess of humour.*

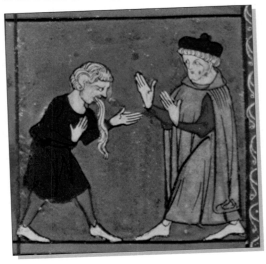

Your doctor might be more of a 'bleeder' though. In order to get your body in balance again, he might want to get rid of your 'bad blood'. Special tools would cut open a vein and bleed you into a bowl. Sometimes, **leeches** were used to suck the blood out of people. You would hope that your doctor was skilled enough to know when to stop before you lost too much blood.

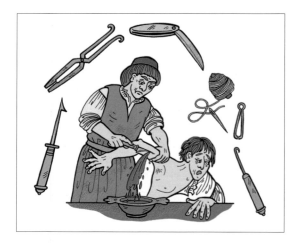

TOP EXAM TIP

For your exam, make sure you know how a medieval doctor might treat illness.

Source F ⮟ *A Zodiac chart. If doctors needed to operate, they would use a zodiac chart to find a safe date. The chart showed a man surrounded by figures to show which constellations (group of stars) were thought to 'rule' different parts of the body. Different parts had to be left alone during the time when its stars were high in the sky!*

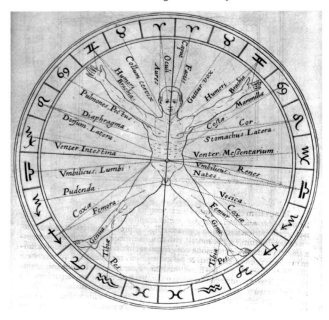

FACT *Hair cut or vein cut, Sir?*

People sometimes visited a **barber-surgeon** to be bled. He was usually a bit cheaper than a doctor and you could have your hair cut at the same time (sharp knives you see!). A barber-surgeon shop was 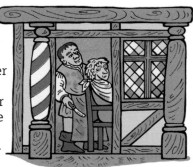 easy to spot because they had a red and white pole outside (red for blood, white for bandages). Some barbers still have poles like these outside their shops today.

FACT *Pilgrimages*

Most people in the Middle Ages believed in God of course so some people would go on a pilgrimage if their doctor's cure wasn't working or they felt they needed that extra bit of holy help. Pilgrims would go to a holy place like the shrine of a saint and pray to God for better health.

FACT *Swallow that? You must be quackers!*

Good doctors were in short supply – and could be expensive. This left things open for **quacks**, people who sell all sorts of potions that are supposed to cure everything. These potions were sold at fairs and by the side of roads ... and usually contained nothing at all to help you to get better!

Source G ▾ *A well-known medieval poem.*

"Against these many kinds of humours overflowing,

several kinds of medicine may be good,

such as diet, drink, hot bath with sweat growing

purging, vomiting and letting blood."

Source H ▾ *An early medieval writer (Isidore, c.620).*

"A doctor must know how to read so that he can understand medical books. He must know how to write and speak well so that he can explain the diseases he is treating. He must have a good mind to investigate and cure the causes of disease. Arithmetic is also important, so that he can count the hours a person is in pain. Music will also be useful for it can be a great help to the sick. Lastly, he must know astronomy so that he can study the stars and the seasons, because our bodies change with the planets and stars."

Source I ▾ *Written in 1380.*

"Doctors possess three special qualifications and these are: to be able to lie without being caught out; to pretend to be honest; and to cause death without feeling guilty."

FACT *Super Salerno*

In the ninth century, a medical school at Salerno in Italy suggested that herbal medicine and prayers were not enough to heal all patients. In the thirteenth century, some disagreed with the great Galen who had said that pus in wounds was good. Two doctors argued that a cut healed quicker if it is closed promptly and pus can't develop. Another doctor, Henri de Mondeville, criticised doctors for getting dirt into patients' wounds – he poured alcohol on wounds to stop them going septic. Hundreds of years later doctors realised that the alcohol was actually killing tiny organisms called germs that were in the wounds!

WISE UP WORDS

- apothecaries   purging   leeches barber-surgeon   quacks

WORK

1 Write a sentence or two to explain the following terms:
   - apothecaries • purging • barber-surgeon
   - quack • theory of the four humours
2 Why do you think doctors bled some of their patients?
3 Is there any evidence that some of the herbal remedies used by medical doctors were successful?
4 Imagine you teach students in a medical school in the Middle Ages. It is your job to welcome them onto the course and provide information on some of the topics they will need to study over the next few years.

   Prepare a leaflet for your students that:
   - outlines the qualities needed for a good doctor (why not read **Sources H** and **I**?);
   - describes the most important topics of study (astrology, herbal remedies, four humours and so on);
   - explains why each of the topics needs to be studied.

CLASSIC EXAM QUESTION

"In the Middle Ages, medicine was still mainly based on Greek and Roman ideas." Explain why you agree or disagree with this statement.

Did they have hospitals in the Middle Ages?

Topic Focus

Make sure you know:
> how hospitals started;
> the difference between the various sorts of 'hospital';
> how important monasteries were.

Exam Focus

> Be able to describe how and why hospitals first developed.

Before studying these pages, think about what a hospital means to us today. What do they do? Why do we go there? What are they like? How are they funded?

If you thought about these questions properly, you would probably come to the conclusion that they are places, largely funded by taxpayers, where people who are ill are looked after and treated. In many ways, we take hospitals for granted today. There probably isn't anyone you know who hasn't set foot in one!

But hospitals haven't always been a feature of everyday life. In the Middle Ages, most people wouldn't have gone near one. After all, being born, being looked after if you were ill and dying were mostly done in people's homes.

So how – and why – did hospitals start?

The word 'hospital' comes from the Latin word *hospitalis*, meaning 'a place for guests'. The idea of a hospital as we know it dates from AD331 when Constantine, the first Christian Roman Emperor, banned the treatment centres of other religions and set up Christian refuges for the sick and needy. They were trying to carry out the teachings of Jesus – which was to help the sick and the poor.

From then on, hospitals popped up all over Europe, most of them paid for by the Church. The oldest working hospital still in use today is the Hôtel Dieu in Paris. It was founded in AD600 (see **Sources A** and **B**).

Source A Hôtel Dieu in Paris.

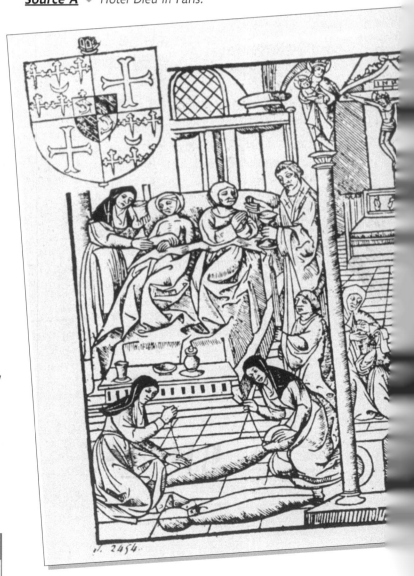

> ## TOP EXAM TIP
>
> *Know how – and why – hospitals first developed.*

Source B ▼ *A description of the work carried out in the Hôtel Dieu in Paris.*

"The work is hard. Quite often, day must become night and night day, so the sick can be cleaned, washed, put to bed, bathed, dried, fed, given drinks, carried from one bed to another, lifted so beds can be remade, personal linen washed out every day in clean water. Every week, between eight and nine hundred sheets can be rinsed in clean water, put into the wash tub, and washed in the River Seine, whether it's freezing, windy or raining, and then hung out to dry in the summer or dried by a great fire in the winter."

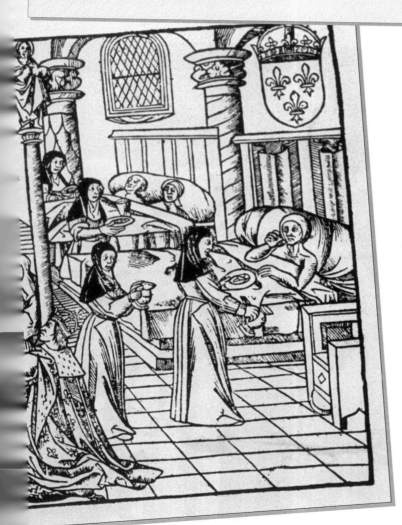

These hospitals varied in size enormously. Some, in cities like Paris or Milan, had hundreds of beds but most took in just ten or twenty patients. And they didn't just look after the sick; they looked after the poor too. Primarily then, they were houses of religion, looking after a patient spiritually as well as physically. Indeed, a doctor might visit occasionally but often just to look after one of the nuns or priests who were caring for you! For a patient, attending lots of church services every day was compulsory. Indeed, the Church paid for 160 new hospitals in Britain between 1205 and 1300.

Our modern view of a hospital is nothing like the view of a person in the Middle Ages. Amazingly, often people who were seriously ill and needed most urgent attention were not allowed in. This was because they would take too much looking after and might stop people praying. So hospitals would be crammed with orphans, cripples, the blind and the elderly. Poor, hungry travellers might stay a few nights whilst poor widows with small children might stay for a few weeks until they found another place to go!

FACT *St Bart's*

St Bartholomew's in London is one of Britain's oldest hospitals. Founded in 1123, it began by concentrating on the care of poor women who were pregnant.

But hospitals weren't the only places that concentrated on looking after the sick and needy – leper houses, almshouses, monasteries and nunneries were also a crucial feature of medical care in the Middle Ages.

TOP EXAM TIP

You need to know what the key features were in monasteries that helped keep the monks healthy.

Leper hospitals

Leprosy was a well-known disease in the Middle Ages. A leprosy victim sees parts of their body decay as large areas of skin, toes and fingers are slowly eaten away. It was viewed as a living death with no cure … and a way for God to punish people for their sins! Lepers weren't allowed to marry, had to wear special clothes and were banned from churches and markets. They even had to ring a bell or shake a rattle to warn people they were near. Special leper houses – or leper hospitals – were built on the edges of some towns to keep the lepers away. They didn't provide any treatment, just a meal and a bed. By the twelfth century, there were nearly 20 000 leper houses in Europe – most of which had disappeared by 1700 as leprosy died out.

Almshouses

These were small houses, often in rows, where the elderly, pregnant women and the weak might stay for a while. Funded by the Church, a priest might be in charge but no real medical treatment was given. Instead, you relied on any herbal remedies the priest might know.

Monasteries

Monasteries became key medical centres in the Middle Ages. Not only did they have copies of books by Greek and Roman writers like Hippocrates and Galen, the monks felt it their Christian duty to look after the sick. Most monasteries (and nunneries) had an infirmary to care for any such monks and an almonry – a building near the monastery wall where poor pilgrims, beggars and the disabled could collect left over food and old clothes. The monks would grow herbs in their garden to make

medicines but they felt that healing was really the work of God, so prayer was the most important part of any treatment of the sick (see **Source E**).

Source C ▾ *From the medieval local laws of Berwick-upon-Tweed.*

> "No leper shall come within the town gates and if one gets in by chance, he shall be put out at once. If he wilfully forces his way in, his clothes shall be taken off him and burnt and he shall be turned out naked."

Source D ▾ *A picture of nuns looking after the sick in their nunnery. Nuns or sisters often attended to the sick – that's why senior nurses in hospitals today are known as 'sisters'.*

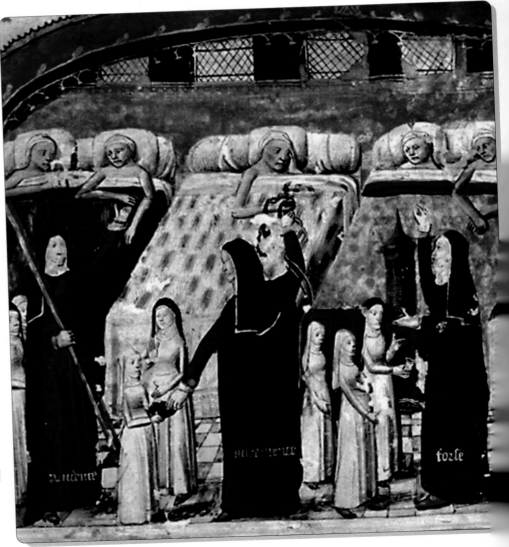

Source E ⬤ *A monastery map of Fountains Abbey, which was founded in 1132.*

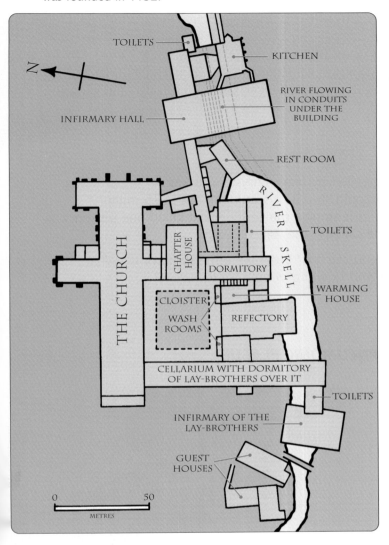

TOILETS
KITCHEN
N
RIVER FLOWING IN CONDUITS UNDER THE BUILDING
INFIRMARY HALL
REST ROOM
RIVER SKELL
CHAPTER HOUSE
TOILETS
THE CHURCH
DORMITORY
WARMING HOUSE
CLOISTER
WASH ROOMS
REFECTORY
CELLARIUM WITH DORMITORY OF LAY-BROTHERS OVER IT
TOILETS
INFIRMARY OF THE LAY-BROTHERS
GUEST HOUSES
0   50
METRES

Source F ⬤ *From the rules of the Hospital of St John, Bridgwater, 1215.*

"No lepers, no lunatics. No people with a contagious disease. No pregnant women, no sucking infants, no intolerable infants – even if they are poor and infirm, and if any are admitted by mistake, they are to be expelled."

Source G ⬤ *The rules for Benedictine monks, AD534.*

"Care for the sick stands before everything. You must help them as Christ would, whom you really help by helping them. Also, you must be patient with them and you will gain greater merit with God. The sick should not be neglected at any single point."

WORK

1 Look at **Source A**. List as many features of the hospital as you can. For example, 'I can see what appears to be nuns caring for patients in bed.'

2 Look at **Source B**. In what ways would the work carried out in the source have made this hospital a healthier place than others?

3 **a** Describe the medieval attitude towards lepers.

   b Why do you think lepers were treated this way?

4 **a** Look at **Source E**. Explain what features in this monastery would help keep monks healthy.

   b Are there any features of this monastery that you think were unhealthy? Explain your answer.

5 Look at **Source F**. Why do you think hospitals made these sorts of rules?

6 **a** Copy out and complete the following chart:

	Purpose	Who went there?	Types of treatment	Who pays for it?
Asclepion				
Medieval hospitals				
Modern hospitals				

   b Which two of the three have the most in common?

Case study: The Black Death

Topic Focus

This case study looks at:
> the symptoms and spread of the Black Death.
> the fear it caused.
> the different reasons people came up with to explain it.

Exam Focus

> Be clear about the impact the Black Death had on the Medieval understanding of health and medicine.

In 1348, the people of England were gripped by fear. A mysterious killer plague was spreading across Europe and nothing could stop it. It would kill about 75 million people in total – 25 million of them in Europe. And as it crossed the continent, it killed one person in every three. No wonder people called it the 'Black Death'!

So what exactly was the Black Death? How could you catch it? What were the symptoms? What did people at the time think caused it? And how did people try to cure it?

How did it kill people?

The Black Death was a plague. The word 'plague' was first used by Galen, the famous Greek doctor, in the second century AD. He used it to describe 'a fast spreading fatal disease'. The Black Death was two different types of plague attacking at the same time. Both still exist today.

PNEUMONIC PLAGUE

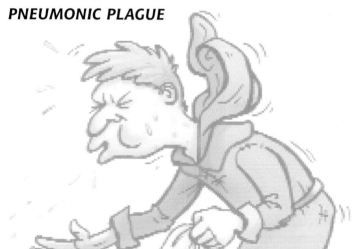

BUBONIC PLAGUE

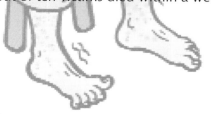

- Came from the germ called Pasteurella pestis.
- The germ lived in the blood of black rats and in the guts of their fleas.
- The fleas would hop off the rats onto humans and bite them … passing on the disease.
- Victims would get a fever and find large boils (called buboes) in their armpits, groin area and behind their ears. They would develop a rash of black and red spots.
- About seven out of ten victims died within a week.

- Caught by breathing in germs or infected air.
- Attacked the lungs. Victims would cough up blood and spray deadly germs as they coughed.
- The victim's breath would smell as their lungs rotted inside them.
- Most victims would be dead within a few days.

Where did it come from?

Source A ▶

The spread of the Black Death. Its origins are unknown, but most historians think the outbreak of the 1300s started in China.

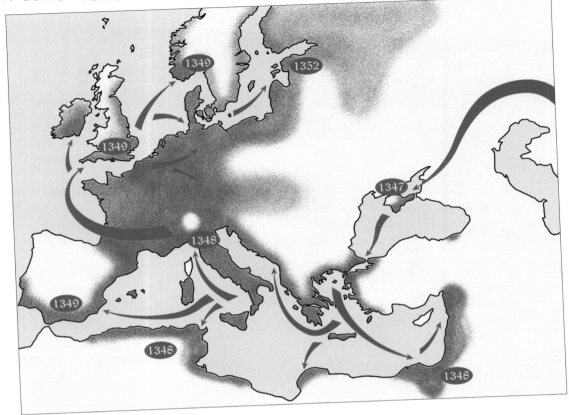

The Black Death arrived in England at the port of Melcombe Regis in Dorset in June 1348. A sailor brought it with him. It had travelled along trade routes from China and India, through the Middle East and then into Europe through Italy. Ships carrying plague-infected people and infected rats landed at ports all over Europe (see **Source A**).

Source B ▾ *Medieval descriptions of the Black Death.*

> i) Lumps in the armpits and the groin. From this, one died in five days.
>
> ii) Fever and spitting of blood. Breathing suffers and whoever has been corrupted cannot live beyond two or three days.
>
> iii) Tumours in the armpits and groin grow as large as apples. Black spots also appear on the arms and thighs.

Source C ▾ *Written by Boccaccio, a famous writer, who was in Genoa, Italy, when the Plague arrived.*

> "In January of the year 1348, three galleys [ships] put in at Genoa. They had come from the East and were horribly infected with the Plague. No one would go near the ships, even though they had a valuable cargo of spices and other goods."

Source D ▾ *From the Grey Friars Chronicle, written by monks in 1348.*

> "In this year at Melcombe [near Weymouth, Dorset], a little before the feast of St John the Baptist [24 June], two ships came into the harbour. One of the sailors had brought with him, from Gascony in France, the disease, and through him the people of Melcombe were the first in England to be infected."

Source E ▾ *A painting called* The Triumph of Death. *It shows us how people at the time viewed the arrival of the Black Death.*

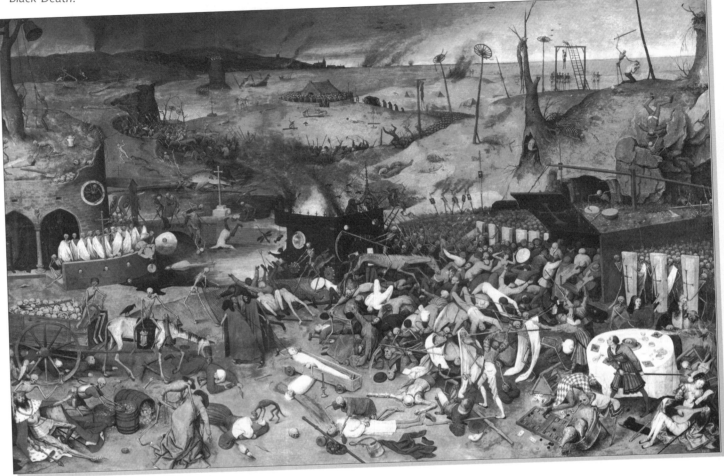

What did people think caused the Black Death?

Doctors didn't know that germs caused disease so looked for other reasons why something so terrible could have happened. **Sources F** to **J** show the different ways in which people at the time tried to explain the cause of the Plague.

Source F ▾ *By an unknown Italian writer.*

"The Plague carried by these cursed Italian galleys was a punishment sent by God. He did this because these galleys helped the unbelievers [Muslims] capture a Christian town."

Source G ▾ *From the* Neuberg Chronicle, *1349. In total, about 12 000 Jewish men, women and children were burnt to death in Germany.*

"In many German cities, Jews were believed to have caused the deaths by poisoning the wells. Many of these unbelievers [Jews], including women and children, were burnt after pleading with them to accept the true faith of Christ. Many Jews were money lenders and people saw a way of wiping out their debts in the flames."

Source H ▼ *Written by John of Burgundy in 1365. Do you think he had read books by Galen?*

"Many people have been killed for the cause of the Plague is not only the corruption of the air, but the corrupt humours within those who die. You should avoid over-indulgence of food; also avoid baths. These open the pores through which poisonous air can enter. Above all avoid sexual intercourse. In cold or rainy weather you should light fires in your chamber. On going to bed, burn juniper branches so that the smoke and scent fills the room.

If the infected blood is in the armpits, blood should be let from the cardiac vein."

Source I ▼ *From a report written by doctors at Paris University in 1348. They had been asked to investigate causes of the Plague.*

"The distant cause

The first cause of the Plague is the position of the heavens. In 1345, at one hour after noon on 20 March, there was a major conjunction of three planets in Aquarius. This caused a deadly corruption of the air.

The near cause

The present Plague has happened because evil smells have been mixed with the air and spread by frequent winds. This corrupted air, when breathed in, penetrates to the heart and destroys the life force.

Hippocrates agreed that if the four seasons do not follow each other in the proper way, then Plague will follow. The whole year has been warm and wet and the air is corrupt."

Source J ▼ *Written by Jean de Venette, 1348.*

"The disease was spread because of **contagion**. If a healthy man visited a Plague victim, he usually died himself."

How did people try to cure the Plague?

Doctors didn't know what caused the Plague so were unable to find a way of curing it and stopping its spread. Some recommended herbal cures to fight the disease, others suggested that you beg God for help. And as the Plague got worse, the 'cures' seemed to get crazier (see **Source K**).

Source K ▼ *Some of the cures suggested at the time.*

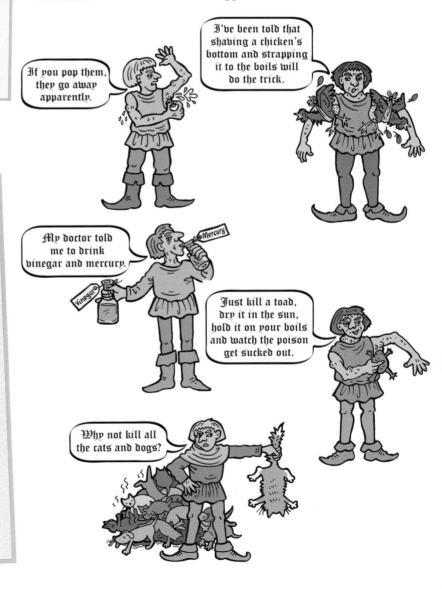

If you pop them, they go away apparently.

I've been told that shaving a chicken's bottom and strapping it to the boils will do the trick.

My doctor told me to drink vinegar and mercury.

Just kill a toad, dry it in the sun, hold it on your boils and watch the poison get sucked out.

Why not kill all the cats and dogs?

Source L ▼ *Some people believed that the Plague was a punishment from God for their sins. They thought that the best way to get rid of your wickedness was to beat it out of you. In Europe, large groups of people, called* **flagellants***, went around whipping themselves hoping that God would take pity on them and stop the Plague!*

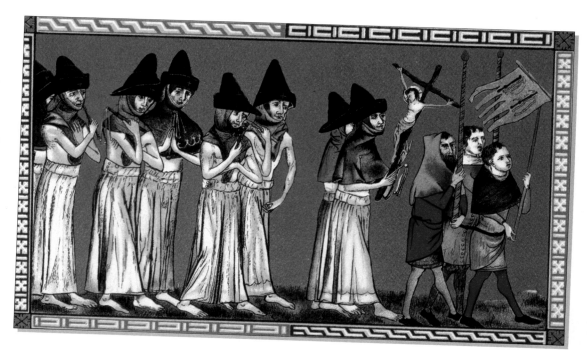

Source M ▼ *These words were scratched on a church wall in Ashwell, Hertfordshire. They read '1349 the pestilence. 1350, pitiless, wild, violent, the dregs of the people live to tell the tale.'*

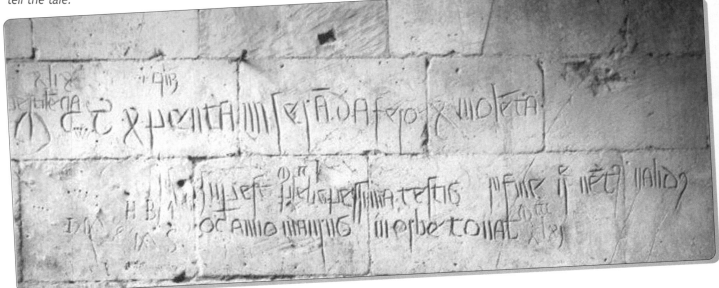

FACT *Germ warfare*

In 1347, an attacking Mogul army catapulted their dead Plague victims into a city they were attacking in order to infect the inhabitants.

TOP EXAM TIP

Make it clear in the exam that you understand how the use of different evidence and sources can lead to conflicting interpretations.

So many people died that graveyards soon filled up and people were left to rot where they fell. By 1353, after spreading up into northern Europe (Denmark, Sweden, Norway), the Black Death died out ... for a while. Five more times it returned before 1400 (although not on the same scale) and it continued to haunt Europe for the next 250 years. As people said at the time, 'the smell of death lies all over this land.'

FACT *Names, names, names*

Today, plagues are usually called **epidemics**. You often hear this word on television if experts are predicting a major health scare. In modern times, one of the worst epidemics was the 'Spanish flu' of 1918–1919. It killed nearly 22 million people in 120 days!

FACT *Rat fact*

In medieval England, rats were a very common sight, feeding on rubbish that piled up in the streets. Rat fleas bit and fed off the rats as well as biting people. And the rats died of the Plague as well.

Source N ▾ *From a modern historian.*

"Conditions were too chaotic for doctors to learn from the Plague. If a doctor tried to learn about the disease by observing plague victims, it would simply increase his chance of dying. In any case, the complex links between rats, fleas, germs and humans could not be understood without two important aids. One was printing, which (from the fifteenth century) enabled people to share their knowledge. The other was the microscope but this wasn't invented until the seventeenth century."

SUMMARY

- People in the Middle Ages believed in magic and the spirits – they thought disease was a punishment from God.

- The theory of the four humours was still accepted, but there was a belief that bad air and smell carried disease too.

- Simple surgery could still be performed but the problems of pain, infection and bleeding still remained. Herbal remedies were still used and bleeding was a common treatment.

- By the end of the Middle Ages there were some hospitals and the rich could visit doctors trained in the ancient ideas of Galen.

WISE UP WORDS

contagion   flagellants   epidemics

WORK

1 a Copy and complete the following table:

	Bubonic plague	Pneumonic plague
How was it caught?		
What were the symptoms?		
How long did it take to die?		

  b Why do you think it was called the 'Black Death'?

  c From what you know about living conditions in villages and towns in the Middle Ages, do you think diseases like the Black Death would have spread very easily?

2 How did the Black Death spread across Europe?

3 Look at **Source E** very carefully. What do you think the artist is saying about the Black Death?

4 Look at **Sources F** to **J**.

  a Make a list of all the different causes of plague you can find in these sources.

  b Why do you think there were so many different explanations of the cause of Black Death?

  c Which source comes closest to the real cause of the Black Death?

5 Look at **Source L**. Why do you think the flagellants behaved as they did?

6 Read **Source N**. According to this source, what hindered medical progress in relation to the plague during the fourteenth century?

7 Design a Black Death poster for 1348. Remember that nobody knew what we know about the causes of plague, so don't include any mention of fleas, germs or rats. Your poster should:

  - warn people about the causes – add pictures to make the message stronger;

  - advise people about the cures available;

  - be eye-catching and informative.

Remember that few people at the time could read. How does this affect the sort of poster you will create?

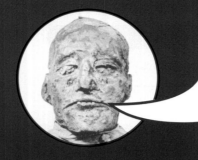

Have you been learning?

TASK 1: TREATING PATIENTS IN ANCIENT EGYPT

Read the two sources carefully. Each one was written in Ancient Egypt about 1500BC and gives instructions about examining poorly patients.

▼ **_Source A_** *Instructions for treating a broken nose.*

"If you examine a man whose nose is disfigured – part of it being squashed in while the other part is swollen and both his nostrils are bleeding, then you shall say: 'You have a broken nose and this is an ailment I can treat.' You should clean his nose with two plugs of linen and then insert two plugs soaked in grease into his nostrils. You should make him rest until the swelling has gone down. You should bandage his nose with stiff rolls of linen and treat him with lint every day until he recovers."

▼ **_Source B_** *Instructions for treating swellings.*

"When you come across a swelling of the flesh in any part of the body of a patient and your patient is clammy and the swelling comes and goes under the finger, then you must say to your patient: 'It is a tumour of the flesh. I will treat the disease. I will try to heal it with fire since cautery heals.' When you come across a swelling that has attacked a channel, then it has formed a tumour in the body. If when you examine it with your fingers, it is like a hard stone, then you should say: 'It is a tumour of the channels. I shall treat the disease with a knife.'"

Once you have read the two sources carefully, identify the evidence that shows the Ancient Egyptians:

a examined their patients;

b diagnosed illness and disease based on their observations;

c could do basic first aid;

d were good at bandaging;

e knew the importance of keeping clean;

f could perform basic surgery.

Use evidence to support each fact.

TASK 2: KNOWLEDGE OF PHYSIOLOGY IN ANCIENT GREECE

Read through **Sources C** and **D**, each written in Ancient Greece in about 500BC.

▼ **_Source C_** *The four humours. From Hippocrates'* On the Constitution of Man *c.500BC.*

"Man's body has blood, phlegm, yellow bile and black bile. These make up his body and through them he feels illness or enjoys health. When all the humours are properly balanced and mingled, he feels the most perfect health. Illness occurs when one of the humours is in excess, or is reduced in amount or is entirely missing from the body."

▼ **_Source D_** *The plague. From Thucydides'* History of the Peloponnesian War *c.5000BC.*

"I shall describe what the plague was like ... at the beginning the doctors were unable to treat the disease because of their ignorance of the right methods. Equally useless were prayers in the temples, consulting the oracles and suchlike."

Once you have read through the sources carefully, identify the evidence that shows the Ancient Greeks:

a believed in the 'theory of the four humours';

b believed in 'balancing opposites';

c believed that an imbalance of humours caused illness and disease.

Use evidence from the sources to support each fact.

TASK 3: MEDICINE IN ROMAN TIMES

Study the following source carefully and then think about the question that follows. A valuable source like this tells us much about opinions on medicine in Roman times.

▼ *Source E* *Pliny's* Natural History *c.AD50.*

"I will not mention many famous doctors like Cassius, Calpetanus, Arruntius and Rubrius. Their annual salaries were a quarter of a million sesterces. When Nero was emperor, people rushed to Thessalus, who overturned all previous theories and when he walked about in public he was followed by as big a crowd as an actor or chariot-driver. Next came Crinas of Massilia, who decided what his patients could eat according to the astrologers' almanacs. There is no doubt that these doctors, in their hunt to gain fame by means of some new idea, did not hesitate to buy it with our lives. Consequently, those wretched quarrelsome consultations at the bedside of patients. Consequently also the gloomy inscription on monuments: 'It was the crowd of doctors that killed me.' Medicine changes every day and we are swept along on the puffs of the clever brains of the Greeks. People can live without doctors (though not, of course, without medicine). It was not medicine which our ancestors hated, but doctors. They refused to pay fees to profiteers in order to save their lives. Of all the Greek arts, it is only medicine which we Romans have not yet practised."

What does the writer, Pliny, tell us about:

a the salaries of doctors in Roman times?

b the status of doctors?

c the abilities of some doctors?

d the general opinion of Greek doctors in Roman times?

TASK 4: SUMMARY

Copy out and complete the following chart, which summarises medical developments from prehistoric to Roman Times. Some of them have been done for you.

	Prehistoric	Egypt	Greece	Rome
Medical problems	Pain, infection, disease, bleeding	Pain, infection, disease, bleeding	Pain, infection, disease, bleeding	Pain, infection, disease, bleeding
Who treated illnesses?	Medicine men, female members of family			Trained doctors, temple priests, female members of family
What did they think caused illness and disease?			The gods, an imbalance of the four humours	
How did they try to prevent and treat illness?		Herbs, basic surgery, charms		Herbs, basic surgery, treatment based on opposites, exercise, public health (sewer system and so on).

TASK 5: QUESTION TIME

Look at these genuine GCSE questions carefully. Why not try to complete them as a revision exercise? In brackets after each question, you will find the pages of this book where there is information that might refresh your memory.

- Explain why the Egyptian were able to make progress in medicine. (pages 12–17)

- In which area of medicine did the Egyptians make the most progress? (pages 12–17)

- 'The Egyptians used natural and supernatural approaches to medicine side by side.' How far do you agree with this statement? Explain your answer. (pages 12–17)

- Explain the theory of the four humours. (pages 20–21)

- Why were the Greeks able to make more progress in medicine than the Egyptians? (pages 18–25)

- Briefly describe the main features of the Romans' public health system. (pages 30–31)

- To what extent was the Roman public health system successful? (pages 30–31)

What do I Revise?

The study of medicine is fascinating … and very detailed. At first it may seem like you have a lot to revise but don't stress out too much about this – you won't be expected to have a detailed knowledge of the whole history of medicine, including all the intricate scientific detail. You are not expected to know about medicine in the same sort of detail as a trainee doctor (you're a history student, after all), but you must understand the following four key areas in order to get the highest marks possible in your exam.

1 Have a basic knowledge of the key medical developments

Your studies will have been divided into a number of different periods of time. Not all exam boards study the same periods, but the most common periods are:

a Prehistoric times

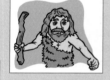

b The ancient world – Egyptians, Greeks and Romans

c The Middle Ages

d The Medical Renaissance

e The nineteenth century

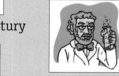

f Medicine in the modern world

You should have a basic understanding of the main medical developments in these periods.

2 Know about the different ideas people had about the causes of disease and examples of different treatments

Throughout history, people have had all sorts of different ideas about the causes of disease. As a result, there has been lots of variety in the way that diseases have been treated. For example:

Ideas about the causes	Treatment
Evil spirits cause disease	Prayers, sacrifices to the gods, use of charms to ward off evil spirits, trepanning to release evil spirits etc.
Disease is related to the balance of the four humours	Keep the humours 'in balance' by bloodletting, purging and so on.
Bad air and rotten smells carry disease and illness	Burn tar in the streets to get rid of the foul air, carry sweet smelling flowers and herbs to cover the smells – and clean the streets to get rid of the stench.
Germs cause disease	Use antiseptic to kill germs, improve public health in general, use antibiotics and introduce vaccination programmes.

Make sure you know about the different ideas people have had about the causes of disease – and examples of the way disease was treated at the time.

The Consequences of Change

Changes in medicine often bring benefits for example: the introduction of antibiotics saved many lives during and after World War Two. Changes that lead directly to benefits are very easy to spot. But there can be disadvantages to change too. For example, when the theory of the Four Humours was first introduced, it was generally accepted that this was the correct way to treat illness. In fact, this incorrect theory influenced the practice of medicine for 1500 years! Sometimes change can have very little impact at all. Improvements in knowledge about human anatomy in Ancient Greece, for example, did not mean that surgery became safer, because there was no antiseptic or anaesthetics!

Continuity

It is important to understand that some ideas and treatments continued for hundreds of years through lots of periods in history. Bloodletting for example, was practiced in Ancient Greece ... and in Stuart London! The ideas of people such as Hippocrates and Galen influenced medicine for centuries.

The Speed of Change

Changes in medicine happen at different speeds in different periods of history. For example, medicine in the modern world has developed rapidly compared with the speed of change in the Middle Ages!

3 Some important ideas and themes about the development of medicine

Regression

A top student must not fall into the trap of thinking that medical knowledge and practice always improves. There have been times when medicine has regressed (got worse). After the Roman Empire collapsed for example, there was a period of decline.

Old and New

It is important to remember that old and new ideas existed side by side in all periods of history. In many periods studied you should have noted that both supernatural and natural theories were used to explain illness.

4 Remember that a wide variety of factors have helped (and sometimes hindered) the development of medicine

a War The use of X-rays in World War One and the development in plastic surgery in World War Two.

b Science and Technology The part played in the advance of medicine by the scientific study of germs in the 1800s and the technology used in modern surgery such as fibre optics, CAT scans and transplant technology.

c Chance Chance has been a key factor in many medical developments. For example in Fleming's discovery of penicillin.

d Government In Ancient Rome the government introduced an advanced public health system, whilst in the twentieth century, the government in Britain introduced the NHS.

e Religion The banning of dissections by the Christian Church meant that knowledge of human anatomy was limited.

f Individuals A key factor is the hard work, intelligence and sheer brilliance of some of the most famous people in medicine – Hippocrates, Galen, Paré, Vesalius, Harvey, Jenner, Lister, Simpson, Snow, Pasteur, Koch, Nightingale and Fleming to name a few.

Remember that advances in medicine usually happen when a combination of these factors come together. The discovery and introduction of penicillin is a classic example of this – individual brilliance, chance, science and technology, government and war all combined in this development.

So what was the 'Renaissance'?

Look carefully at **Sources A** and **B**. **Source A** is a drawing of the human body from the Middle Ages. **Source B** is a drawing of the human body sketched during a period of history that has now become known as 'the Renaissance'.

It seems obvious that the person who drew **Source A** didn't really know much about the human body at all. It is also obvious that the person who drew **Source B** had studied the human body in graphic detail.

So what exactly was the Renaissance? And how did it lead artists to make incredibly detailed and accurate drawings like the one shown in **Source B**?

The Renaissance was a period that began in the 1400s. The invention of the printing press made books cheaper than ever before – and they were a lot easier to buy. As more books were printed, more people wanted to read. There were new books on fishing, hunting, chess, travel and different types of religion. But people also began to read the old books written by the Ancient Greeks and Romans who lived before Christ. They soon found that the Greeks and Romans knew a lot more than anyone had realised. Across Europe, writers, sculptors, doctors, mathematicians, scientists and architects started to realise that some of their current ideas were wrong and there were better ways of doing things. They began to ask questions and experiment with new ideas. Scientists carried out new experiments, explorers set out for new lands, doctors tried new treatments and artists used new methods to make their paintings more lifelike than ever. For years, people had accepted that the Bible had all the answers to their questions. Now, educated people no longer wanted the Church to tell them what they should think. They wanted to find out for themselves.

As people's interest in ancient knowledge was rekindled, many likened the experience to being 'reborn' ... and the word 'renaissance' is an Italian one meaning 'rebirth'.

One of the most famous 'Renaissance men' was a painter named Leonardo da Vinci. He was a scientist, mathematician, engineer, inventor, musician and poet too. In order to paint the human body correctly, he cut up dead bodies to see how they worked. In total, he made over 30 dissections – and at a time when this was a very dangerous thing to do. The Church had banned dissection of human bodies because they believed that people needed their whole body in their life after death.

Through his experiments, Leonardo worked out how the human eye worked and was the first to study a human embryo in detail. Indeed, his research – and the sketches that went with it – were so good that doctors examined his work before starting an operation (see **Source B**)!

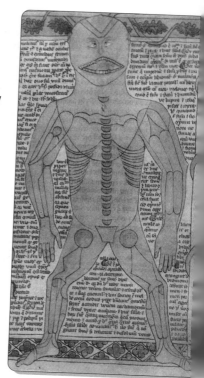

**Source A** ▸ _A medieval drawing of the human body._

Source B ▶

Drawings by Leonardo da Vinci. Like many 'men of the Renaissance', Leonardo didn't believe all he read. He dissected bodies himself in order to make accurate drawings.

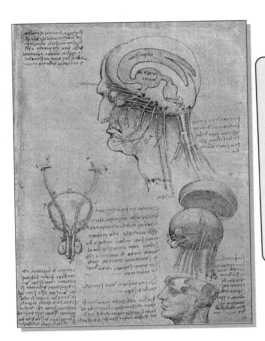

Source C ▾ *Advice given by Leonardo da Vinci to art students in 1519.*

"The painter who has a knowledge of the sinews, muscles and tendons will know exactly which sinew causes the movement of a limb ... he will be able to show the various muscles in the different parts of his fingers ... you will need three dissections to have a complete knowledge of the arteries, three more for the membranes, three for the nerves, muscles and ligaments, three for the bones and cartilages. Three must also be devoted to the female body..."

TOP EXAM TIP

Make sure you know how key features of the Renaissance would affect the development of medicine.

Source E ▾ *What caused the Renaissance?*

New lands – the discovery of the Americas in the late 1400s showed the value of finding new things, rather than sticking to old ideas. New foods and medicines were also brought back from this 'new world'.

New learning – a scientific method of learning began. This involved conducting an experiment, collecting observations and then coming to conclusions. Soon scholars began to question old established beliefs – and this was vital for the development of medicine.

Why was there a rebirth?

Artists – a new desire to paint the body in more detail led artists to study the body more carefully. This was connected to an improved knowledge of anatomy.

New weapons (like gunpowder) – meant soldiers got new types of wounds ... which doctors had to find new methods to deal with.

The printing press – allowed new ideas to spread quickly around Europe ... and allowed old textbooks to be re-discovered.

WORK

1 **a** What is meant by the word 'renaissance'?
   b How did the invention of the printing press help the Renaissance?

2 **a** How did Leonardo da Vinci and Michelangelo help the progress of medicine?
   b Why do you think the first accurate drawings of the human body were made in the Renaissance?

3 Look at **Source E**. How did:
   i) the introduction of gunpowder
   ii) the discovery of new lands
   iii) new scientific methods
   help the progress of medicine?

A renaissance in medicine: what were the new discoveries?

Topic Focus

▸ Did the medical discoveries made during the Renaissance have much impact on health care?

Exam Focus

▸ You will need to know why Vesalius, Paré and Harvey are important.

The development of medicine during the Renaissance period was led by three men. Their names were Andreas Vesalius, Ambroise Paré and William Harvey. Each was a key individual in the development of their chosen areas – anatomy (how the body is studied), surgery (how patients are operated on) and physiology (how the body works). As you read their stories, you must decide how important each person was. Think how Vesalius changed the way the human body was studied, how Paré changed battlefield surgery and what Harvey discovered about blood.

Andreas Vesalius (1514–1564)

1

Born in Brussels in 1514.

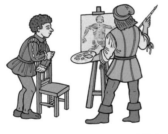

He studied medicine in France and Italy where he met artists who were studying skeletons and cutting up bodies to make their paintings more realistic.

2

At Padua University in Italy, students were encouraged to have new ideas.

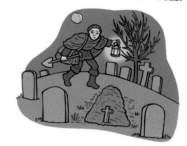

He robbed cemeteries and acquired the bodies of executed criminals to dissect.

5

Vesalius worked on his own book about anatomy.

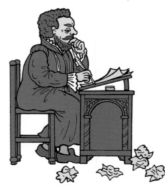

The Fabric of the Human Body was published in 1543. It contains fantastically detailed sketches of the human body drawn by some of the world's finest artists.

3

In 1537, he became Professor of Surgery at Padua University.

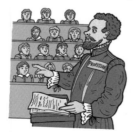

He told his medical students to perform dissections for themselves, stating that 'our true book of the human body is man himself'.

4

Vesalius was a very popular teacher.

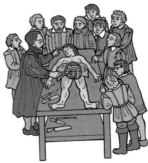

Eager students crowded into his lectures to watch what he did and listen to what he said.

6

Vesalius' book caused a sensation.

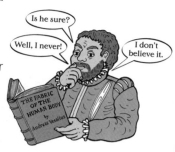

Vesalius showed that the famous Greek doctor Galen was wrong in some of the things he wrote. For hundreds of years, doctors had believed that his ideas about the human body were entirely accurate!

7

Doctors had been taught to believe that Galen was right. Now Vesalius was doing the unthinkable.

As soon as some of Galen's ideas were proved wrong, others became keen to carry out more and more experiments to test Galen's theories for themselves.

* Galen's theory ~ Right or Wrong?
* The human breastbone has seven segments ~ <u>Wrong</u> it has three!
* The human jawbone is made up of two bones ~ <u>Wrong</u> it is made up of one
* Blood passes from one side of the heart to the other through holes in the septum <u>Wrong!</u> The septum is too thick, it must move another way.

8

One of Vesalius' theories proved very controversial indeed.

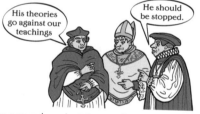

Vesalius argued against the traditional view that women have more ribs than men. He showed that both sexes have the same number. This angered Church authorities because they taught that God had taken a rib from the first man, Adam, and used it to make the first woman, Eve!

9

Vesalius was criticised again and again by the Church.

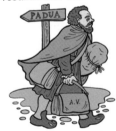

Upset by the criticisms, Vesalius left Padua and spent the rest of his life working as a doctor for Emperor Charles V of Spain. He died in 1564.

TOP EXAM TIP

Note how Vesalius' fame depended on factors not related to medicine – a good artist and the invention of the printing press.

FACT *Paracelsus*

Another influential man of the Renaissance was Swiss scientist Paracelsus (1493–1541). He searched Europe and the Middle East for knowledge and challenged many existing ideas about disease. He disagreed with Galen by arguing that disease attacks from the outside rather than from within and introduced the now familiar idea that doctors should look for specific symptoms of a disease and then prescribe a specific cure.

Source A ▸ *An illustration from Vesalius' book.*

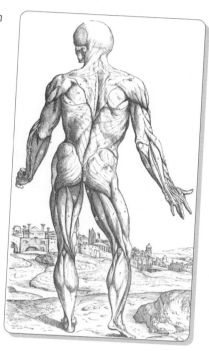

The work of Vesalius was important in the development of medical knowledge because he corrected many of the mistakes made by Galen and others. For centuries, doctors had been taught that there was no need to learn any more about the human body because Galen had provided all the answers. Now Vesalius had shown the value of dissecting human bodies to find out exactly how they work. He said doctors needed to test Galen's theories and carry out new experiments rather than believe his theories without question.

Source B ▸ *Vesalius showing the muscles of the human arm.*

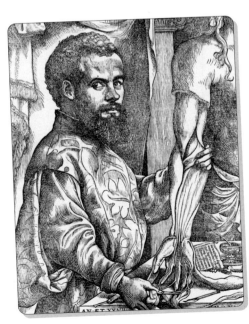

Ambroise Paré (1510–1590)

Born in 1510, Ambroise Paré started work as a hospital surgeon with his brother in Paris at the age of 13. At 25, he became an army surgeon and spent the next 20 years travelling around with the French army treating all sorts of terrible wounds. His ideas changed battlefield surgery forever.

So, if we were able to travel back in time to the 1500s, what would an interview with Ambroise Paré have sounded like? Despite the fact that Paré would probably have been too busy saving soldiers' lives, if by the chance he found the time to talk to us, an interview with the most famous army surgeon of all might have gone a bit like this:

Interviewer: Ambroise Paré, you are the most famous surgeon in Europe – how did it all start?

Paré: I was born in a small village in France and becoming a surgeon was a bit of a family tradition. When I was a teenager, I was apprenticed to my brother, a barber-surgeon. I then worked as an assistant surgeon at the Hôtel Dieu, the main hospital in Paris. I became an army surgeon in 1536, travelling with the French army, treating sword and gunshot wounds.

Interviewer: Are battlefields *really* as dangerous as you might imagine?

Paré: Most definitely. Soldiers face swords, arrows, daggers, pikes and axes … and since the invention of gunpowder, they face the dangers of guns, muskets, bullets and cannonballs too. The injuries suffered are horrendous – and the conditions we have to work in are pretty grim too!

Interviewer: Tell us about these conditions.

Paré: Battlefields are dirty places. Explosions churn up the ground and mud, blood and bullets fly all over the place. Gunshot wounds are a new and devastating wound. Surgeons were meant to follow the theories laid down in a book called *Of Wounds in General* by Jean de Vigo, which says you must pour boiling oil on a gunshot wound to 'kill' the poisonous injury.

Interviewer: You say you were *meant* to follow this procedure!

Paré: Well, yes, a few years after beginning my battlefield work, I started to use other methods. During one battle, our boiling oil ran out. Instead, I used a mixture of my own, made out of egg yolk and cold oils. I rubbed the ointment into the wound and covered it with clean bandages.

Interviewer: And did it work?

Paré: I worried about those patients so much that night that I could hardly sleep. I was convinced that the patients I had treated with boiling oil would be well – and the others treated with my own mixture would be dead.

Interviewer: And were they?

Paré: Not at all. The men treated with my own mixture were sitting up in bed looking comfortable. Their wounds were getting better. But it was a different story for the men treated in the 'old' way. Their wounds were red and swollen and they cried out in pain. A few were dead. From that day on, I vowed never again to use boiling oil to treat gunshot wounds – and I have taught other surgeons to do the same!

Interviewer: A real success story. We hear you try to stop bleeding with new and improved methods too.

Paré: On the battlefield, many men lose limbs – or get so badly injured that we have to chop off a hand or foot because we cannot save it. The usual treatment to stop the bleeding is to press a red-hot iron – called a **cautery** – onto the stump. The idea is to seal the blood vessels by burning them shut!

Interviewer: The pain must be excruciating!

Paré: That is exactly what I thought – so I sought a better way to stop the bleeding.

Interviewer: So what did you do instead?

Paré: I began using silk threads – or **ligatures** – to tie off the veins and arteries in the leg or wrist. It took a long time – 53 ligatures were

needed for a thigh amputation for example
– but it proved to be a very effective way to
stop bleeding.

Interviewer: Did you face any opposition to
your new ideas?

Paré: Absolutely. Surgeons respect tradition,
the established way of doing things, and my
ideas took a long time to catch on. But
luckily I live at a time when some surgeons
and doctors are prepared to try new things.
In wartime, you *have* to experiment and
'think on your feet' – it's the only way to
save lives!

Interviewer: So what's next for you?

Paré: I have just completed a book called
Works on Surgery in which I outline my
theories. I have written it in my native
language, French, but I hope it will be
translated into many other languages and
inspire surgeons around Europe. I will also
continue to develop my highly technical
artificial limbs. They can be used by the
injured soldiers whose limbs I have removed!

FACT *British surgeons*

- William Clowes (1540–1604) – copied Paré's
work. Surgeon to Elizabeth I and worked at St
Bartholomew's Hospital. Wrote a famous book
on gunshot wounds.

- John Woodall (1556–1643) – wrote a popular
book called *The Surgeon's Mate*, which detailed
all the surgical instruments a ship should have
before setting out to sea.

- William Cheselden (1688–1752) – introduced a
90-second operation for the removal of gall-
bladder stones.

- Richard Wiseman (1622–1676) – surgeon to
Charles II. Realised it was a mistake to copy
old ideas and was impressed by writers in other
countries who were experimenting with new
ideas. He wrote two long books on surgery,
which agreed with many of Paré's methods (but
Wiseman himself still used hot oil on bullet
wounds, unlike Paré!).

When Paré retired from the army, he went on to
work for three successive French kings. By then, he
was the most famous surgeon in Europe and his
work encouraged other medical men to try out new
techniques and challenge old methods.

FACT *Infection*

Despite the less painful method of using ligatures
instead of a red-hot iron to stop bleeding, Paré was
still criticised heavily because many of his patients
still died. What surgeons didn't know at the time
was that his patients were dying because germs
were infecting the wounds, carried on the dirty silk
thread used to sew up wounds. It would be several
hundred years before a usable antiseptic would be
developed to make surgery safer from infection.

Source C ▶ *A
nineteenth-
century painting
of Paré tying
ligatures on a
wounded
soldier.*

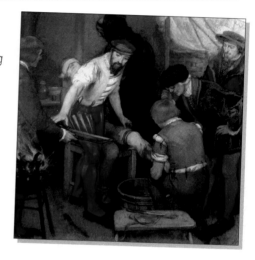

Source D ▼ *Some of Paré's artificial limbs from his book*
Works on Surgery. *Paré never went to university and was
looked down on by other surgeons as a result. In 1585, he
published another book,* Apology and Treatise, *to defend
his ideas.*

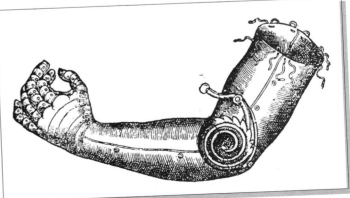

Pause for thought

How did each of these factors help Paré's work and the spread of his ideas:
i) war   ii) Paré's brilliance
iii) the printing press?

FACT *Thomas Sydenham*

In the late 1600s, Thomas Sydenham became one of the most famous doctors in London. He was known as the 'English Hippocrates' because he favoured the close observation of patients and their symptoms. He always tried to use common sense cures and didn't like to interfere with the patient too much by bleeding or purging them. He is even attributed as the first man to discover scarlet fever.

TOP EXAM TIP

Make sure you understand that people were important both in their lifetime and long after because their work often made the work of others possible.

William Harvey (1578–1657)

Born in Kent, England, in 1578, William Harvey went to Cambridge University to study medicine aged 16. Six years later, he travelled to the great medical school in Padua, Italy, to complete his education. Back in London, he soon gained a reputation as a superb doctor and in 1609, began working at St Bartholomew's Hospital in London. He was also surgeon to King James I and Charles I. By now, he had become fascinated with blood … and how it moves around the body.

Harvey took a very scientific approach to medicine, carrying out dozens of experiments and making detailed notes. At the time, most doctors still believed the old Greek idea that dated back over 1000 years. The old theory was that new blood was constantly being manufactured in the liver to replace blood that was burnt up in the body like fuel. This idea had been challenged by a number of doctors but no one had totally discredited the theory. Harvey's experiments showed that the idea was wrong. He found that the heart acts as a pump, circulating the SAME blood all

the time. He showed that the heart pumped blood to the body through arteries and the blood returned to the heart through veins.

He proved this by:

- cutting up lots of frogs (their hearts beat slowly and he could see how they worked);
- cutting up human beings (usually the bodies of hanged criminals) to see how their bodies worked;
- pushing thin wires down veins (to help to show that there are valves in the veins that make blood flow around the body);
- measuring the amount of blood moved by each heart beat and calculating how much blood is in the body.

Source E ▾ *A drawing from Harvey's book showing his experiment to demonstrate the function of the valves in the veins. a) The upper arm was bandaged to restrict the flow of blood and make the valves (G, O, H) visible. b) A finger was pushed along a vein from one valve to the next in a direction AWAY from the heart (O to H). c) The vein between O and H emptied of blood … and stayed empty because valve O didn't allow blood to flow back.*

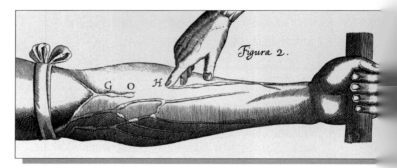

Harvey published his ideas in 1628 in a book called *On the Movement of the Heart and the Blood in Animals*. But there was a gap in his explanation. He believed that arteries were connected to the veins by tiny capillaries … but he couldn't see them with the naked eye. As a result, his ideas were considered a little too 'crazy' for the time and he actually lost patients (see **Source F**). It was only in the 1660s, a few years after his death, that an Italian doctor, Malpighi, used a new microscope to prove the capillaries did actually exist (as Harvey predicted). In fact, in Harvey's lifetime, his discoveries made little difference to the treatment patients received – it was only years later that his theories made their impact (see **Source G**).

WISE UP WORDS

- cautery   ligatures

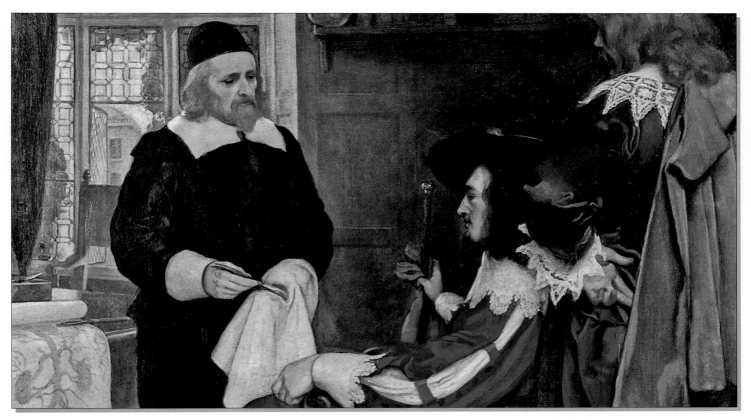

Source F ▼ *A friend of Harvey's recorded this in his diary.*

"I have heard him [Harvey] say that after his book came out he lost a great many patients because it was believed he was 'crack-brained'."

Source H ▲ *William Harvey explaining the working of the heart to King Charles I.*

Source G ▼ *A modern historian.*

"Harvey's discovery is one of the most important in the history of medicine. It gave doctors a new map of how the body worked. Without it, surgeons today would not be able to carry out blood transfusions or any complicated internal surgery."

CLASSIC EXAM QUESTION

a) Choose one of the following medical pioneers: Andreas Vesalius, William Harvey, Ambroise Paré. Summarise in 50 words what he did?

b) Which of the medical pioneers contributed most to improved medical knowledge during the Renaissance. Explain your answer.

WORK

1 Copy and complete the following chart:

Name	What discovery did he make?	How did he make his discovery (observation /experiment /by chance)?	Which old ideas did he challenge?	Did he improve people's health immediately or in the long term?
Andreas Vesalius				
Ambroise Paré				
William Harvey				

2 Look back at the diagram (**Source E**) on page 72. How did some of these key features of the Renaissance help Vesalius, Paré and Harvey in their work? For example, artists who were able to draw accurate drawings of the human body helped Vesalius because he was able to include correctly detailed pictures of his new discoveries in books.

Case study: Ring-a-ring o' roses

Topic Focus

▸ Read this topic and consider whether people in the 17th century understood plague any better than people did in the 14th century when facing the Black Death.

Exam Focus

▸ Make sure you can compare reactions to the Black Death with those to the Great Plague.

Look at **Source A**. Workmen digging foundations for a new building in London found this mass of skeletons just below the surface of the ground. It is a plague pit – one of many mass graves dotted around the capital. These pits contain the remains of some of the 70 000 or more people who died in the summer of 1665 during the Great Plague.

So why were people buried in pits rather than in their local churchyard? How did people catch the Plague and where did it come from? What measures did Londoners take to avoid the Plague? Did it spread outside London? And what did the Great Plague teach doctors about the treatment of illness … and what do their efforts tell us about their knowledge of health and medicine in the seventeenth century?

Source A ▾

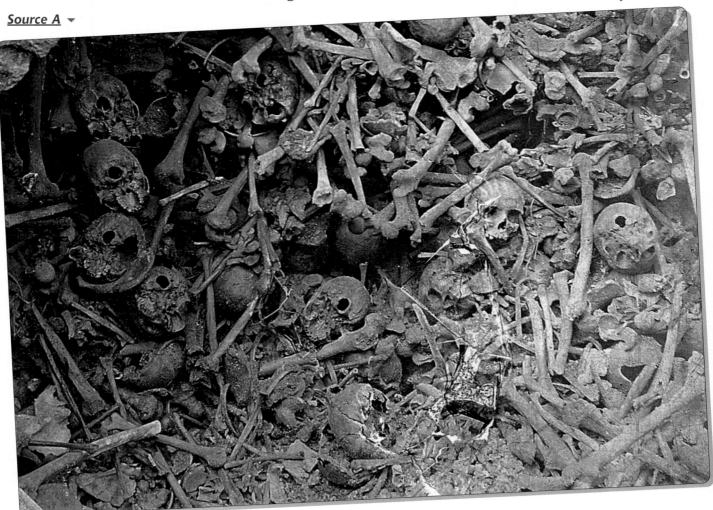

You should remember your studies of the Black Death, a deadly plague that swept through Europe in the fourteenth century. Plague continued to strike Britain at regular intervals throughout the 1400s and 1500s. Then, in 1665, London was hit by the worst outbreak for hundreds of years. Over 70 000 people died … and there were only just over 400 000 people living in London at the time. Study carefully **Sources B** to **G**. They show what was done at the time to stop the Plague spreading. From the information, you can work out how people thought the Plague was spread.

Source B ▼ *Special orders issued by the Mayor of London in an attempt to stop the spread of Plague.*

- Any house containing a Plague sufferer has to be sealed up for 40 days until the person is dead or better.

- The door of the house has to be marked with a red cross and the words, 'Lord, have mercy upon us'.

- 'Searchers' are to be appointed to examine each corpse for 1p per body to find out the cause of death.

- Public entertainments are to be stopped.

- All dogs and cats are to be caught and killed; the dog catcher is to be paid about 1p for each animal.

- Fires are to be lit in the streets.

- Bodies are to be buried after dark.

Source C ▶ *Three drawings from a Plague broadsheet (a kind of news leaflet) printed in 1665. In picture 1, look for: the examiners checking each house; dogs being killed; men taking away rubbish (householders had to keep their houses clean); a fire in the street (some believed bad air was responsible for the Plague – so fires were lit to purify the air). In picture 2, look for: the mass grave; the dead woman who has dropped down by the road; birds dropping from the sky – they must have flown into some bad air and been killed! In picture 3, look for: the searchers (with the long poles) examining people who were ill or had died; the coffin ready for the dead person on the left; the doctor on the right giving medicine to the patient in the bed.*

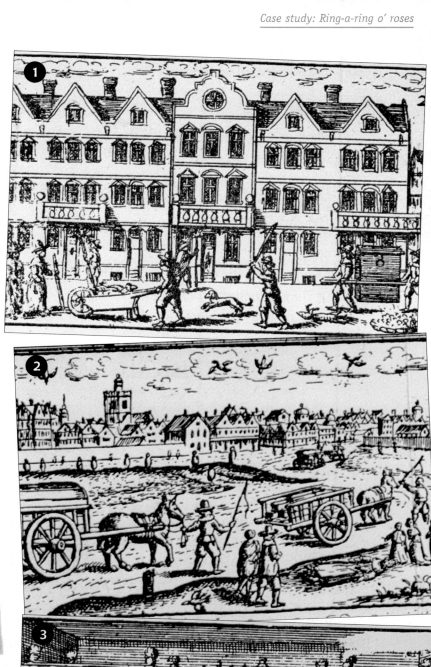

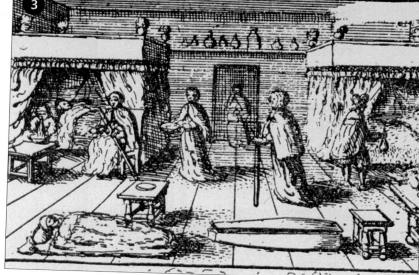

Source D ▼ *In 1722, Daniel Defoe (who was born in about 1660) wrote* A Journal of the Plague Year.

"When anyone bought a joint of meat in the market, they would not take it from the butcher's hand, but took it off the hooks themselves. On the other hand, the butcher would not touch the money, but had it put in a pot full of vinegar. The buyer always carried small money, so that they might take no change."

Source E ▼ *From* In Search of History 1485–1714.

"From a letter written in August:

The sickness increases. There are many who wear amulets [charms] made of toad's poison which, if there is any infection, it raises a blister, which a plaster heals, and so they are well… [In September] It is increasing. Friend, get a piece of gold. An Elizabethan coin is the best. Keep it always in your mouth when you walk out or any sick persons come to you: you will find strange effects of it for good in freedom of breathing, if you lay with it in your mouth without your teeth, as I do."

WISE UP WORDS

- bubonic   Bill of Mortality

Source F ▼ *Plague doctors wore costumes like this when they visited victims.*

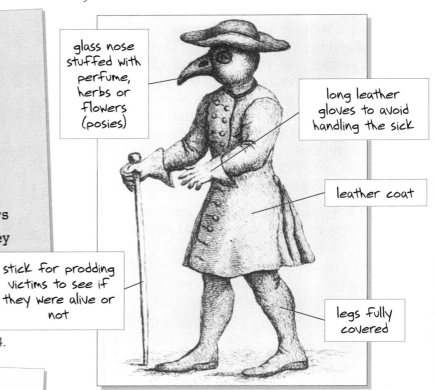

glass nose stuffed with perfume, herbs or flowers (posies)

long leather gloves to avoid handling the sick

leather coat

stick for prodding victims to see if they were alive or not

legs fully covered

Source G ▼ *People spent a fortune on crazy cures like this one. Today, it is easy to laugh at them but try to imagine how scared people must have been at the time. They were obviously willing to try anything. The 'sore' the writer of this strange recipe refers to is one of the boils that were a common symptom of the Plague.*

Recipe for the Plague

Wrap in woollen cloths, compel the sick party to sweat which if he does, keep him there until the sores begin to rise. Then apply a live pigeon cut in half or a plaster made of the yolk of an egg, honey, herbs and wheat flower.

There are different kinds of plague, each with a different cause. Historians cannot quite agree on the type of plague that hit London in 1665 but most think it was probably **bubonic**. It gets its name from the 'buboes', or huge round boils which appeared in a victim's armpit or groin. Other symptoms included fever, shivering, dizziness, vomiting, aches and pains, a rash of black and red spots and diarrhoea.

Historians think that plague-infected rats and fleas brought the disease to England aboard boats bringing goods from Holland. The rats and fleas soon carried the disease all around the filthy streets of London. Towns such as Sunderland, Newcastle and Southampton were also hit by the Plague as people fled there to escape the horrors of London.

In 1665, people didn't understand what caused the Plague or how to treat it properly. Many thought it was caused by bad air, others said it was sent by God as a punishment; some believed cats and dogs spread it. Today, we know most of the answers. We know that the Plague was a germ that lived in the guts of fleas. The fleas were carried in the fur of the black rat. A single fleabite was enough to kill a person. Fortunately, for the people of England, the autumn of 1665 was very cold and by December, the Plague was almost over. It claimed a few thousand victims in 1666 but killed nowhere near as many as in the summer months of the previous year.

FACT *Smoking in school ... allowed!*

The boys at Eton School in Surrey were punished if they *didn't* smoke tobacco! Can you think of a reason why a teacher would want their pupils to smoke?

Source H ▼ *Searchers would check each dead body to work out the cause of death. Each week the number of dead and their cause of death were written on a* **Bill of Mortality***. This one covers 12–19 September 1665.*

Source I ▼ *A nursery rhyme, said to be about the Plague and its symptoms. The 'roses' refer to the rash of red and black spots on a victim's body; the posies refer to the flowers many carried around with them to ward off bad smells that some thought caused the Plague. A'tishoo refers to the sneezing fits many victims had and 'we all fall down' speaks for itself!*

> " *Ring-a-ring o' roses,*
> *A pocketful of posies,*
> *A'tishoo, A'tishoo,*
> *We all fall down.* "

WORK

1 Look at **Source B**.
   a Write down in order those you think might actually prevent the Plague from spreading. For each one, explain why you made your choice.
   b Many people disobeyed these orders. Why do you think they did this?

2 Look at **Sources D** and **E**.
   a Make a list of the different ways people tried to avoid the Plague.
   b Do you think any of these measures would have made people safer from the disease?
   c In your opinion, do you think people in the seventeenth century understood the Plague better than people did in the fourteenth century at the time of the Black Death? Think about:
      • their thoughts on how you caught the disease;
      • their ideas for preventing it;
      • their ideas on how the Plague spread.

3 Look at **Source H**.
   a What is a Bill of Mortality?
   b How many people died of the Plague that week?
   c How many people died and were buried 'in all' during the week?
   d Work out what percentage of people were killed by the Plague during this week.
   e What evidence is there that the Plague was increasing during this particular week?
   f Why do you think there were so few babies christened this week?

CLASSIC EXAM QUESTION

Between the Black Death and the Great Plague was there much progress in people's ideas about disease?

Curing King Charles

Topic Focus

▶ Make sure you know how King Charles II was treated
... and why he was looked after in this way.

At 8:00am on 2 February 1685, King Charles II suddenly fainted. It was soon clear that he was seriously ill. A dozen doctors crowded round him, trying to save his life. This was their chance to prove themselves as great doctors. If they saved him they would be richly rewarded. Fail and their King dies ... and they didn't want the blame for that!

Like all doctors, they had a choice of treatments. And because their patient was so important, one of the doctors (Sir Charles Scarborough) wrote down the treatments given to the King. The descriptions of the things done to Charles in his final days give us an amazing insight into the state of medical theory in the late seventeenth century. After all, his doctors would be trying all the latest ideas ... wouldn't they? So how was the King treated? On what ideas did his doctors base his treatments? And, did the medical treatment help to heal the King's pain ... or did it help to finish him off?

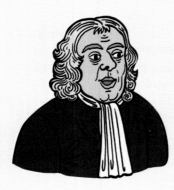

2 February 1685

His Majesty felt some unusual disturbance of the brain, soon followed by loss of speech and convulsions.
— We opened a vein in his right arm and drew off about 16 ounces (425ml) of blood.
— We then had a conference and prescribed three cupping glasses to be applied to his shoulders. About 8 ounces (212ml) of blood were withdrawn.
— So as to free his stomach of all impurities, we gave an emetic (to make him vomit).
— Soon after, we gave (laxative) pills so as to drain away the humours. Further we supplemented this with an enema.
— To leave no stone unturned, his hair was shaved and blistering agents were applied all over his head.

3 February 1685

We ordered sacred tincture (a liquid medicine) every six hours. Meeting at noon we considered it necessary to open both jugular veins and draw off about 10 ounces (300ml) of blood. At this point the King complained of a pain in the throat and a gargle of barley water and syrup was prescribed. Further it seemed most desirable that his bowels should be kept continuously relaxed by giving two ounces of sacred tincture.

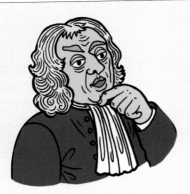

4 February 1685

It seemed advisable to prescribe a mild laxative. As His Majesty's condition got worse during the night, we prescribed the following: 40 drops of spirit of human skull and a half of Julep (a sweet alcoholic drink).

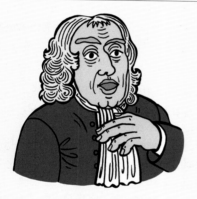

6 February 1685

Alas, after an ill-fated night, His Majesty's strength seemed exhausted. In spite of every treatment attempted by doctors of the greatest skill, he was seized quite unexpectedly by a mortal distress in breathing [and died].

So King Charles II died! He was 54 years old. Some time later, it was discovered that the King had a kidney disease. The last thing Charles needed was bloodletting. In fact, losing blood is one of the worst treatments a kidney patient should receive. His doctors actually shortened his life!

CLASSIC EXAM QUESTION

Use your knowledge of the Great Plague and the death of Charles II to explain how little the Renaissance changed about:

a) ideas about the cause of disease and

b) methods of treatment.

Source A ▼ *A picture of Charles II touching people to cure a common skin disease of the time known as 'King's evil'. Charles (and many of his doctors) believed he could heal them because he was their King, put on the throne by God. Between 1660 and 1682, Charles touched over 92 000 people with skin diseases! His own surgeon, Richard Wiseman, even wrote how he had witnessed people being cured by the King (yet still treated people for 'King's evil' himself – and cured them – with medicine and a good diet!).*

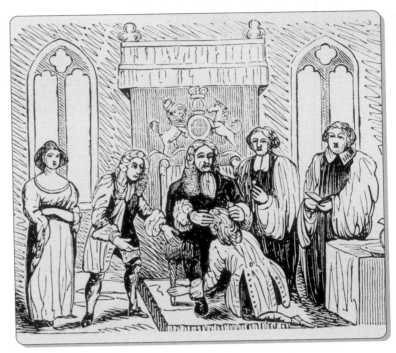

WORK

1 Look at **Source A**.
  a How did King Charles cure 'King's evil'?
  b Why do you think so many people visited King Charles?
  c By the mid 1700s, people stopped visiting the monarch to be cured of King's evil. What does this tell us about people's faith and its connection to medicine during this time?

2 King Charles was treated in a variety of ways. Make a list of each treatment and then, next to each idea, explain:
  i) what the theory behind the treatment was;
  ii) whether the idea was a supernatural or natural one;
  iii) whether the treatment was a new or old idea.

The Medical Renaissance · **79**

Did giving birth get any easier?

Topic Focus

▶ This topic will help you understand the sort of problems faced by both mother and child during childbirth, and why these problems persisted.

Exam Focus

▶ You should be able to understand and describe what medical progress there was, and why, in dealing with childbirth.

Even today, with all our modern technology, safety equipment and standards of hygiene, childbirth is an incredibly dangerous time for both the baby and their mother. It has always been a dangerous time!

King Henry VIII, for example, a person who could afford the best medical care, saw seven of his first wife's eight babies die! Another of his wives (Jane Seymour) died just after childbirth herself. In fact, childbirth remained one of the main causes of death amongst women of childbearing age well into the 1900s.

So why was childbirth such a dangerous time? Who actually helped women to give birth? And did the developments of the Medical Renaissance make childbirth any easier?

What was known about childbirth?

The Ancient Egyptians, Greeks and Romans knew a lot about the female reproductive system. But during the Middle Ages, much of the knowledge was 'lost' and little progress was made. The obstacles to progress were religious. In the West, the barriers to progress were put up by the Church; in the Arab world, by Islam. Both religions considered it wrong for male doctors to examine the female reproductive organs. As a result, female patients were looked after by other females (perhaps a relative or the local wise woman). And it was highly likely that these women had absolutely no medical training or qualifications at all. So childbirth was incredibly 'hit and miss' – sometimes a mother survived, sometimes she didn't … and it was the same for the baby (see **Source A**).

Source A ▶ *From the diary of Alice Thornton, aged 27, in 1652. Women often got pregnant when they didn't want to, as there was no reliable contraception.*

6 August 1652

About seven weeks after I married, it pleased God to give me the blessing of conception. The first quarter I was exceeding sick in breeding, after which I was strong and healthy, I bless God. Mr Thornton had a desire I should visit his friends. I passed down on foot a very high wall … Each step did very much strain me … The skilled my sweet infant in my womb … who lived not so long as we could get a minister to baptise it … After the miscarriage I fell into a most terrible shaking fever… The hair on my head came off, my nails on my fingers and toes came off, my teeth did shake, and ready to come out and grew black…

Alice Thornton, my second child, was born in Hipswell near Richmond in Yorkshire the 3rd day of January 1654.

Elizabeth Thornton, my third child, was born at Hipswell the 14th of February, 1655. [This child died 5th September 1656.]

Katherine Thornton, my fourth child, was born at Hispwell … the 12th June, 1656.

On the delivery of my first son and fifth child at Hispwell the 10th of December, 1657 … the child stayed in the birth, and came crosswise with his feet first, and in this condition continued till Thursday morning … at which I was upon the rack in bearing my child with such exquisite torments, as if each limb were divided from the other… but the child was almost strangled in the birth, only living about half an hour, so died before we could get a minister to baptise him…

17 April 1660

It was the pleasure of God … to bring forth my sixth child … a very godly son … after a hard labour and hazardous. [The child died two weeks later.]

19 September 1662

I was delivered of Robert Thornton … it pleased the great God to lay upon me, his weak handmaid, an exceeding great weakness, beginning, a little after my child was born, by a most violent and terrible flow of blood, with such excessive floods all that night that my dear husband, and children and friends had taken their last farewell.

23 September 1665

[She was pregnant once more.] I being terrified with my last extremity, could have little hopes to be preserved this time … if my strength were not in the Almighty … It pleased the Lord to make me happy and a goodly strong child, a daughter, after a exceeding sharp and perilous time. [The child died on 24 January.]

Christopher Thornton, my ninth child, was born on Monday, the 11th of November 1667. It pleased his Saviour to deliver him out of this miserable world on the 1st of December, 1667.

Did the Medical Renaissance help women?

From the 1500s onwards, books were published on childbirth that included information about special chairs used to help mothers to give birth and about the correct positioning of the baby. In Vesalius' book *The Fabric of the Human Body*, he included the first accurate description of the reproductive organs of a woman. Leonardo da Vinci too drew detailed pictures of the human embryo. But the increase in knowledge didn't help women too much. Very few women came into contact with a doctor before the 1600s. In fact, it was most unusual for a man – even the husband – to be present at the birth. Pregnant women were usually helped by other women, perhaps a midwife who had helped other local births. They might call on the wise woman from the village too who might know a few herbal remedies to dull the pain and fight infection after the birth. Still, many women and their babies lost their lives during childbirth (see **Source B**).

Source B ▼ *From a seventeenth-century gravestone in a churchyard.*

REST IN PEACE

Nineteen years a maiden
One year a wife
One hour a mother
And so I lost my life.

'The doctor is here now'

In the late 1600s, men began to take over the medical care of pregnant women, particularly in richer households. They may have attended a course on childbirth run by William Smellie in Edinburgh or William Hunter in London. They tried out new techniques for giving birth, including the use of new medical equipment. Women were even encouraged to go to a hospital rather than give birth at home.

However, the changes didn't necessarily bring about improvement. **Forceps** – a special tool that fits around the baby's head – were developed to free a baby's head if it was stuck. But these could do great damage to mother and baby if not used properly … and they were never sterilised or washed properly.

There wasn't much development in the field of pain relief either and, as a result, the number of deaths remained very high. Even well into the nineteenth century, one in five mothers died in childbirth … and one in six births resulted in the death of the baby.

Source C ▼ *A diagram from the 1700s showing forceps in action.*

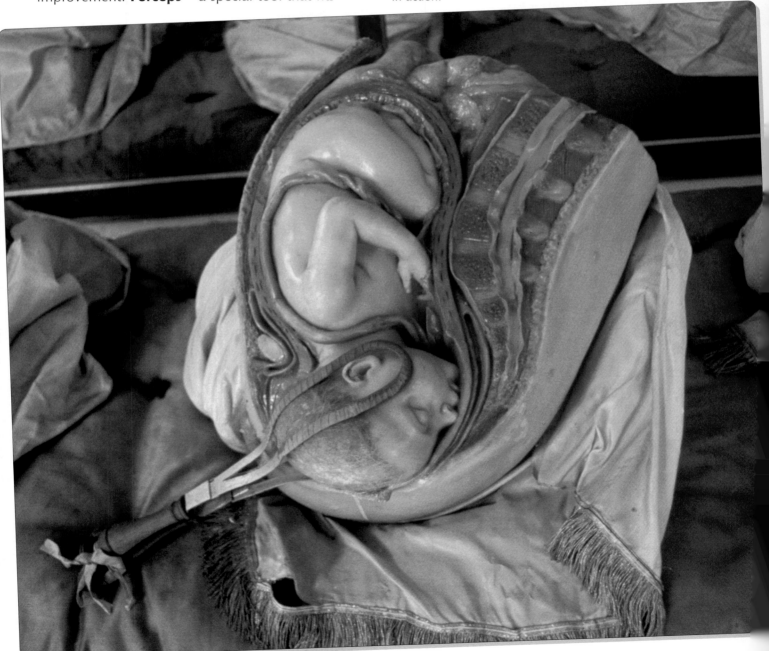

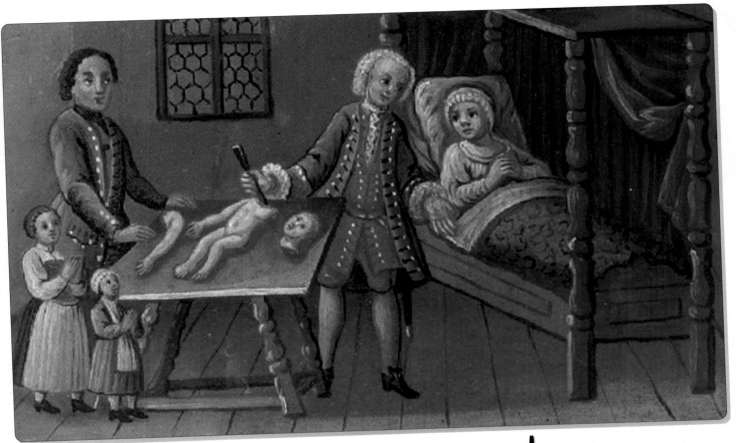

Source D ▲ *An engraving from the 1700s showing the disastrous results of the use of forceps.*

SUMMARY

- The Renaissance period of history saw some monumental developments in medicine.

- Vesalius, Harvey and Paré proved that some of the ancient theories were wrong – but their work had little impact immediately. However, their work inspired others and became the foundation on which later scientists built their discoveries.

- By the end of the eighteenth century, scientists knew germs existed but not that they caused diseases.

- Only simple surgery could still take place.

WORK

1 **a** Why was little progress made in the care of pregnant women in the Middle Ages?

   b Did the Medical Renaissance improve the care of pregnant women? Think about your answer carefully.

2 Read **Source A**.

   a How many times was Alice Thornton pregnant?

   b How many of her babies lived to the age of one?

   c How many years of her life were taken up with childbearing?

3 Look at **Source B**. How effectively does this source show the dangers of childbirth during this period?

4 **a** What are forceps?

   b In what ways did forceps sometimes make childbirth even more dangerous?

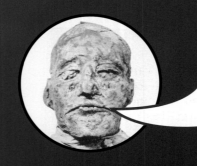

Have you been learning?

TASK 1: THE MEDIEVAL DOCTOR

The following passage appears in Geoffrey Chaucer's *Canterbury Tales* of 1387. It describes a medieval doctor ... and tells historians a lot about medicine in medieval times.

▼ **Source A** A medieval doctor. Chaucer, *Canterbury Tales* c.1387.

"A Doctor too emerged as we proceeded.
No one alive could talk as well as she did
On points of medicine and of surgery
For, being grounded in astronomy
He watched his patient's favourable star
And, by his Natural Magic, knew what are
The lucky hours and planetary degrees
For making charms and effigies.
The cause of every malady you'd got
He knew, and whether dry, cold, moist or hot;
He knew their seat, their humour and condition.
He was a perfect practicing physician.
All his apothecaries in a tribe
Were ready with the drugs he would prescribe
And each made money from the other's guile
(They had been friendly for a goodish while)
He was well-versed in Aesculapius too
And what Hippocrates and Rufus knew
And Disocorides, now dead and gone,
Galen and Rhazes, Hali, Serapion.
In blood-red garments, slashed with bluish-grey
And lined with taffeta, he rode his way;
Yet he was rather close as to expenses
And kept the gold he won in pestilences."

1 Now list the wide range of different ideas and superstitions used by doctors in the Middle Ages. You should be able to list at least five, for example:

'According to Chaucer, a medieval doctor believed that the stars and planets had an impact on health and fitness. In the source, Chaucer writes that the medieval doctor was "grounded in astronomy, he watched the patient's favourable star...".'

2 In your opinion, what was Chaucer's opinion of the doctor?

TASK 2: TREATING ILLNESS

Read through the following sources carefully, then think about the question that follows.

▼ **Source B** Johannes de Mirfield on a medicinal bath from *Flowers of Bartholomew* c.1375.

"Here is a bath which has proved to be of value. Take blind puppies, gut them and cut off the feet; then boil in water, and in this water let the patient bathe himself. Let him get in the bath for four hours after he has eaten, and whilst in the bath, he should keep his head covered, and his chest completely covered with the skin of a goat, so he won't catch a sudden chill."

▼ **Source C** Guy de Chauliac on reducing swelling. From *Surgery* c.1350.

"Bleeding and purging, cordials and medicinal powders can be used. The swellings should be softened with figs and cooked onions, peeled and mixed with yeast and butter, then lanced and treated like ulcers."

▼ **Source D** John of Gaddesden on toothache. From *English Rose* c.1314.

"When the gospel for Sunday is read during the service of the Mass, let the man hearing Mass sign his tooth and his head with the sign of the Holy Cross and say the Lord's Prayer. It will keep him from pain and cure the tooth, so say trustworthy doctors."

What do these sources tell us about the treatment of disease in the Middle Ages?

When writing your answer, think about:

- the effectiveness of the treatments;
- the reasoning behind some of the treatments – why did they do some of these rather strange things?

TASK 3: 'A BLOODY TALE'

Two thousand years ago, Galen, the most famous doctor in Rome, said that blood passes through the septum (a thin tissue that separates sections of the heart) where it is pumped to the muscles and then burned up. In 1628, William Harvey correctly concluded that blood circulates round the body (which he correctly described) and it is <u>not</u> burned up ... it just keeps circulating. The gradual discovery of the circulation of blood is a good example of how medical knowledge can build up over time.

Study the chart carefully.

TASK 4: QUESTION TIME

Look at these genuine GCSE questions carefully. Why not try to complete them as a revision exercise? In brackets after each question, you will find the pages of this book where there is information that might refresh your memory.

- Describe the state of public health in medieval towns. (pages 46–47)
- In what ways were Roman towns healthier than medieval towns? (pages 30–31)
- Describe the main features of Vesalius' work. (pages 68–69)
- Explain how Paré was helped in his work by chance. (pages 70–71)
- Who is more important in the history of medicine – Vesalius or Harvey? (pages 68–69 and 72–73)

Name	Date	Who	Contribution to debate	Influence
Start point – Galen	c.200	Doctor in Rome	Said blood **passes through the septum**, and the heart pumps it to the muscles, where it is burned up.	Main authority for 1500 years.
Ibn an Nafis	c.1250	Persian doctor	Said blood does **not** go through the septum, and is pumped past the lungs.	Muslim doctor, not known in Europe.
Leonardo da Vinci	d.1519	Artist	Made detailed drawings of the anatomy of the heart.	Drawings not discovered until 1850.
Vesalius	1543	Professor at Padua	Said blood does **not** pass through the septum.	Well-known anatomical textbook.
Servetus	d.1553	Italian preacher	Said blood **does** go through the septum, and is pumped past the lungs.	No effect – burned as a heretic.
Columbo	1559	Professor at Padua	Said blood does **not** go through the septum, and is pumped past the lungs.	William Harvey read his book.
Caesalpino	1571	Professor at Padua	First used the word 'circulation' in relation to blood, but could not explain the process.	William Harvey did not know of his work.
Fabricius	1603	Professor at Padua	Discovered valves in the veins only allow the blood to go one way.	William Harvey's teacher at university.
William Harvey – End point	1628	London doctor	Proved that blood circulates round the body, and described how it happened.	

Now identify or write about:

a an error in understanding that lasted many years;

b the importance of education and training;

c the importance of printing and books;

d a discovery that remained undetected in Europe.

Give 'em what they want!

Your guide to understanding how to answer different types of questions

GCSE History courses require you to learn tons of fascinating facts, loads of interesting stories, dozens of famous names and lots of key dates. Your teacher will work incredibly hard to help you work on ways to remember as much of this as you can. But a GCSE History course is not just about filling your head with all this knowledge ... you actually have to sit an exam or two as well! But the exam is not simply designed to test what you can remember, it is aimed at testing your skills as a historian too. As a result, the exam questions themselves, and the way they are worded, are designed to test these skills. So it is vital that you understand exactly what each type of question requires you to write in order to get the best marks possible. Look carefully through the list of key words that most commonly appear in exam questions. Remember, giving the examiner what they want is one of your keys to success.

State...

Write the main points briefly.

Define...

Give the meaning.

Summarise...

Bring together the main points into a short sharp paragraph or two.

Contrast...

Look for differences.

Compare...

Are the things very similar (alike) or are there important differences? You might be asked which is best, and why?

Outline...

Choose the most important parts or aspects of a topic. Generally speaking, ignore the minor detail and concentrate on the 'bigger' points.

Justify...

Write down the main reasons to support an argument or action.

Discuss...

Write about the important aspects of the topic. Think whether there are two sides to the question or argument and consider both sides.

Describe...

This means you have to write in detail about the event, situation or discovery for example. Write down lots of key facts.

Evaluate...

Use your knowledge or the information in front of you to judge the importance or success of something.

Explain why...

Make something very clear, giving lots of detail.

Have a go yourself!

Understanding what the examiner actually wants you to write should lead to a much better grade. Try some of these questions yourself:

- Describe the state of public health in Roman towns.
- Compare public health in a Roman town with a medieval town.
- Explain how the Renaissance helped the progress of medicine.
- Summarize the work of either Vesalius, Paré or Harvey.
- State what is meant by The Theory of the Four Humours.

The smallpox story

▸ The examiner will want you to show that you know exactly how Jenner discovered vaccination.

One of the biggest killer diseases before 1800 was smallpox. This highly infectious virus passed from one person to another by coughing, sneezing, or in some cases, touching. The first symptoms were a fever and headache. A rash then turned into a mass of huge, pus-filled blisters covering the body. When the blisters dropped off, they left deep scars. And it could kill too. In the 1700s, smallpox killed more European children than any other disease … and there was no known cure. So when Edward Jenner, a country doctor from Gloucestershire, found a way of protecting people against it, it was hailed as one of the greatest medical triumphs ever. So how did Jenner make his breakthrough?

FACT *Smallpox victims*

Smallpox has claimed many royal victims. They include Ramases V of Egypt (died 1157BC), Mary II of England (died 1694), Peter II of Russia (died 1730), Louis XV of France (died 1774) and Luis I of Spain (died 1742), two emperors of Japan (both died 548) and the Inca Emperor Huayna-Capac (died 1526).

Source A ▾ *A child with smallpox in Gloucester Infirmary, 1896.*

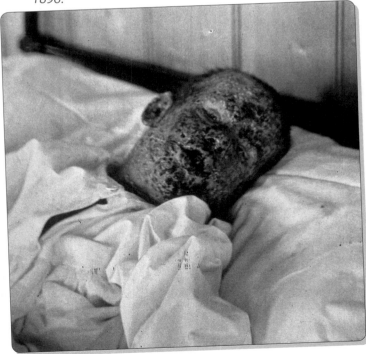

1 In parts of China, people had been using a basic form of **inoculation** for many years.

They scratched pus from a smallpox victim into their skin. They didn't realise it but this gave them a small dose of the disease and allowed their body to build up a resistance against future attacks.

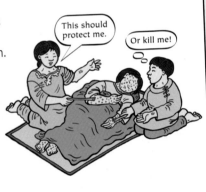

2 Inoculation was being used in Turkey too. In 1717, Lady Mary Wortley Montague lived there.

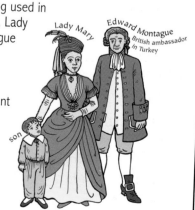

Mary wrote an account to a friend in Britain of how local Turkish people inoculated themselves.

3 Mary had only just survived a smallpox attack herself. She was keen to get her children inoculated.

In 1721, Mary's children survived a dreadful smallpox outbreak. News spread fast — even King George I had his grandchildren inoculated.

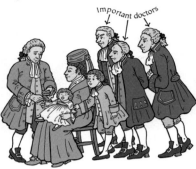

Important doctors

4 Smallpox inoculations became big business. Robert Sutton and his son Daniel were two of the best-known 'inoculators'.

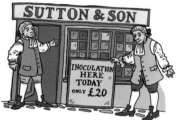

SUTTON & SON

INOCULATION HERE TODAY ONLY £20

They inoculated nearly 14 000 people in 1764 … and made a fortune. But only the rich could afford it.

5 But there were problems with inoculation, aside from its cost.

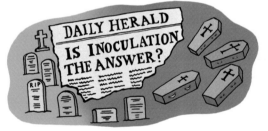

DAILY HERALD
IS INOCULATION THE ANSWER?

Sometimes it gave people a strong (instead of small) dose of smallpox — which killed them! And any inoculated person could continue to spread it to others.

6 The inoculation theory of avoiding smallpox was well known when Edward Jenner became a doctor in the 1770s.

Jenner studied in London with John Hunter, the greatest surgeon of the time. Hunter encouraged his students to use their powers of observation to carry out new experiments.

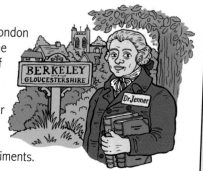

BERKELEY GLOUCESTERSHIRE

Dr Jenner

7 Jenner heard that milkmaids who caught cowpox (a similar, but milder version of smallpox) from cows never seemed to catch the deadly smallpox.

Some people — like farmer Benjamin Jesty from Dorset — deliberately gave themselves cowpox. None of them caught smallpox.

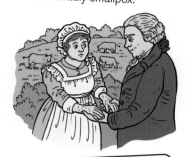

8 In 1796, Jenner decided to carry out an experiment. He used a poor local boy and gave him a dose of cowpox germs.

James Phipps

Worried mother

Six weeks later, he gave the boy some smallpox germs — 'but no disease followed'.

9 Jenner carried out the experiment 23 times. Only then did he conclude that 'cowpox protects the human from the infection of the smallpox'.

His findings were rejected by the Royal Society so he published his research himself. He called his technique '**vaccination**' because the Latin word *vaccinus* means 'from a cow'.

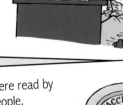

10 Jenner's findings were read by many important people. Parliament gave Jenner £30 000 to open a vaccination clinic.

By 1803, doctors were using Jenner's technique in America. In France, Napoleon had all his soldiers vaccinated! In 1852, the British government made smallpox vaccination compulsory.

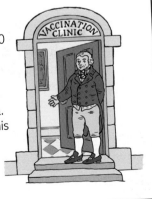

VACCINATION CLINIC

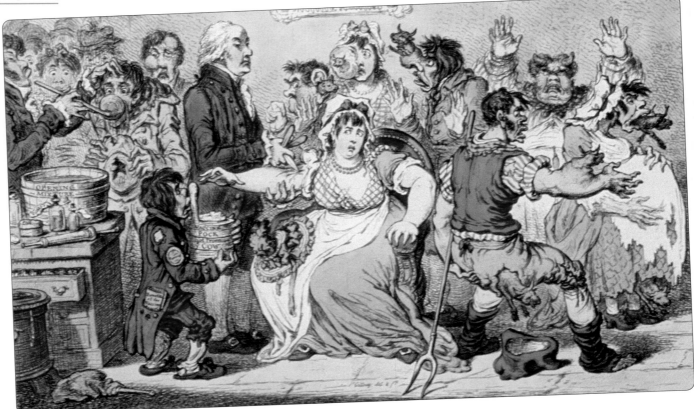

Source B ▲ *A cartoon by James Gillray called* The Cow Pock *or* The Wonderful Effects of the New Inoculation. *In your opinion, does this painting support Jenner's vaccination programme or does it poke fun at it?*

Jenner faced lots of opposition to his findings. Some people simply didn't like anything new – and Jenner wasn't a fashionable London doctor with a big reputation to push forward his findings. Others thought the idea too bizarre to believe. Jenner couldn't actually explain how it worked and this made it difficult for others to accept vaccination. Also, many doctors who were making money out of inoculations didn't want to lose that work!

Pause for thought

To be entirely accurate, the word 'vaccination' started out life referring to the small doses of cowpox given to prevent the onset of smallpox. And no other diseases acted in the same way as cowpox did to smallpox, leading some people to call vaccination a bit of a 'dead end'. Over time, however, vaccination has come to mean the injection of dead or weakened organisms which give the body resistance against all sorts of disease.

Source C ▼ *Extract from Jenner's medical notes, 1798.*

"Case 16   Sarah Nelmes

Sarah Nelmes, a dairy maid near this place, was infected with cowpox from her master's cows in May 1796. A large sore and the usual symptoms were produced.

Case 17 James Phipps

I selected a healthy boy, about eight years old. The matter was taken from the [cowpox] sore on the hand of Sarah Nelmes and it was inserted on 14 May 1796 into the boy by two cuts each about half an inch long. On the seventh day he complained of uneasiness, on the ninth he became a little chilly, lost his appetite and had a slight headache and spent the night with some degree of restlessness, but on the following day, he was perfectly well.

In order to ascertain that the boy was secure from the contagion of the smallpox, he was inoculated with smallpox matter, but no disease followed. Several months later he was again inoculated with smallpox matter but again no disease followed."

Source D ▾ *Deaths from smallpox in England and Wales, 1848–1920. In 1980, the World Health Organization announced that there had been no cases anywhere in the world for the previous two years. The announcement followed a worldwide mass vaccination programme. It seems today that the only place where smallpox exists is in scientists' laboratories!*

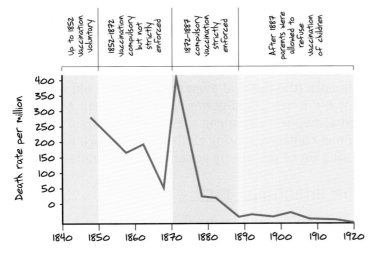

FACT *And now for the science bit!*

Cowpox is a very similar disease to the more deadly smallpox virus. If a person is infected with the low-risk cowpox virus, their body creates antibodies to fight the germs. The antibodies 'lock on' to the cowpox germs and kill them. These antibodies remain in the body ... so when cowpox germs (or anything similar – like smallpox) strike again, the antibodies attack and kill them very quickly. The body is now immune.

So how important was Jenner?

Jenner was not the first to use cowpox as a vaccine against smallpox. Benjamin Jesty, a Dorset farmer, infected his family with cowpox and a local doctor, Doctor Trowbridge, heard about Jesty's idea and tried it out on his own sons. They all avoided smallpox. But neither of these men publicised their ideas. So the reason Jenner appears in this book in great detail is because he showed the willingness to follow the idea up and publish his findings.

TOP EXAM TIP

Jenner is a classic example of a person who knew <u>how</u> to do something ... but did not know why it worked!

It was Jenner's genius to work on the idea, test it scientifically and push hard to publish his investigations. Despite never actually understanding how vaccination worked, Jenner realised that his findings could further our knowledge of disease and save lives. It goes to show though that it is rare for just one person to be associated with a major medical breakthrough.

WISE UP WORDS

- inoculation   vaccination

TOP EXAM TIP

Jenner is a good example of how new medical ideas were often opposed. Make sure you understand why this was the case.

WORK

1 Think carefully.
  a What, in theory, is the difference between inoculation and vaccination?
  b What were the disadvantages of inoculation?

2 **a** Write down the role played in the smallpox story by:
    i) Lady Mary Wortley Montague
    ii) Robert and Daniel Sutton
    iii) Doctor Trowbridge
  b So inoculation and even vaccination existed before Jenner. Does this mean he is not important? Explain your answer carefully.

3 In the 1700s, milkmaids were sometimes called 'pretty maids'. How is this connected to smallpox?

4 Look at **Source B**. This cartoon was published when Jenner's work became well known.
  a What attitude did the people who published this cartoon have?
  b Why do you think they felt like this?

5 How were:
  i) chance
  ii) scientific experiments and investigation
  iii) individual brilliance
  iv) government action
  each responsible for the discovery and development of a smallpox vaccine?

How did scientists discover that germs cause disease?

Topic Focus

▸ Read these 6 pages to understand the importance of Pasteur in proving his "germ theory", and how he applied it to vaccination.

Exam Focus

▸ Make sure you can list the reasons why Pasteur and Koch were important in advancing medical knowledge about germs.

Infectious diseases like measles, chicken pox, mumps, influenza (the flu) and even the common cold are passed from one person to another. They are caused by tiny life forms called germs. Very, very small germs are called viruses. Direct contact – touching or sneezing on someone – can mean the germs (and then the disease) can pass from one person to another. Even indirect contact – sharing clothing or utensils, for example, can pass some diseases between people. The passing on of disease by contact is called contagion.

Discovering 'germs'

The idea that tiny creatures might cause disease – and pass it around – is not a new one. Roman doctor Marcus Terentius Varro suggested this theory 2000 years ago but couldn't prove anything because he couldn't see these minute living things with the naked eye. What he needed, of course, was a microscope!

Instead, most people continued to think that the gods caused disease in some way – usually as a punishment for doing something wrong! This theory survived well into the Middle Ages.

The microscope

In 1677, a clock maker from Holland, Anthony van Leeuwenhoek, made a very basic microscope. To his amazement, he found tiny creatures moving about in nearly all of the things he placed under his new invention. He found them in water droplets, pepper, food, animal intestines and even human poo! He even found them in scrapings he took from his own teeth. He called them 'animalcules' and published his findings.

So 'animalcules' (later called 'germs') had been discovered … but there was still no link made with disease!

'The infectious mist'

By the 1800s, the **miasma** theory of disease had become very popular. Miasma – an 'infectious mist' – rose out of decaying matter such as wood, rubbish, water, soil or animal remains and mixed with the air. This 'bad air' drifted around on the wind, infecting people with all sorts of diseases.

Miasma got the blame for all sorts of outbreaks, illnesses and epidemics over the years too. Many blamed miasma for the Great Plague of 1665, for example. You may even remember that some people carried around 'a pocketful of posies [flowers]' to sweeten the air and overcome the 'bad air' that they felt might cause them harm.

So where did the 'germs' fit into this muddled medical mess?

'Spontaneous generation'

Scientists using microscopes kept identifying germs in the blood of sick people. But they didn't realise it was the germs that had made each person ill. Instead, they thought that the disease somehow caused the germs – not the other way round! This was known as the theory of **spontaneous generation** – the idea that living things – germs, maggots, flies – could appear as if by magic if the conditions were right.

But some people began to question this theory. One of them was a chemist named Louis Pasteur.

Louis Pasteur

Pasteur was born in France in 1822. He studied chemistry and biology, taking charge of science at Lille University in 1854. And it was his reputation as a top chemist that first led one of Lille's top wine producers to go to Pasteur for help…

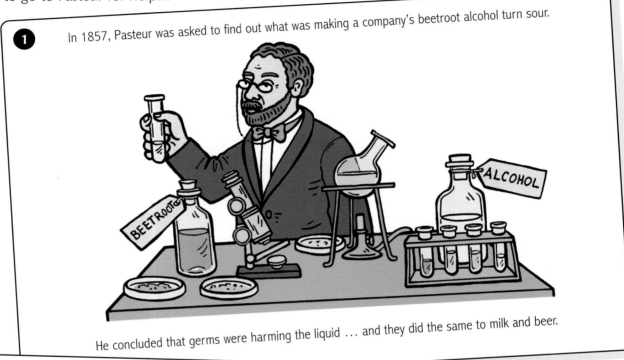

1 In 1857, Pasteur was asked to find out what was making a company's beetroot alcohol turn sour.

He concluded that germs were harming the liquid … and they did the same to milk and beer.

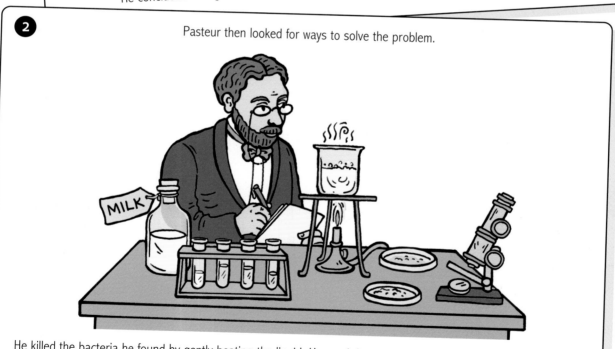

2 Pasteur then looked for ways to solve the problem.

He killed the bacteria he found by gently heating the liquid. He used the same technique with beer and milk. He had invented a process called 'pasteurisation' — it was a huge step forward in keeping liquids free from germs and safe to drink.

3 Pasteur was now convinced that the germs were coming from the air around him. He tried to prove the idea of 'spontaneous generation' wrong.

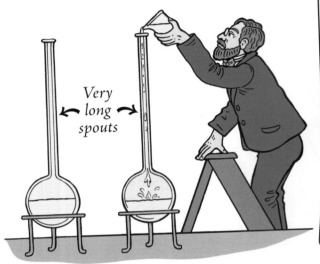

Very long spouts

He used two glass containers and put liquid in each. Then he boiled it to kill all the germs.

4 He heated the spout of one flask until it started to melt. Then he bent it into a curvy shape.

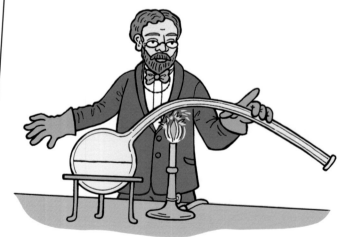

Pasteur claimed that the liquid in the flask with the bent tube would last for years and not turn sour.

5 Pasteur said that the bend in the spout would stop the movement of air.

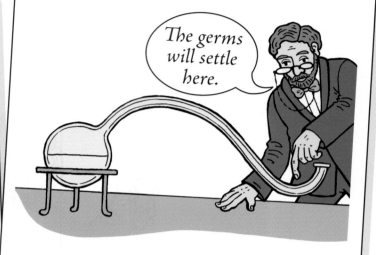

The germs will settle here.

He said that the germs in the air would settle in the lowest part of the curve and wouldn't reach the liquid.

6 Pasteur argued that the liquid in the other flask would soon go bad.

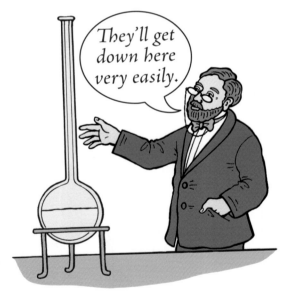

They'll get down here very easily.

He said that the straight spout would allow germs to get to the liquid easily.

TOP EXAM TIP

After the theory of the Four Humours, the Germ Theory is the next major turning point in the history of medicine. You need to know why!

7 Everything Pasteur said was correct.

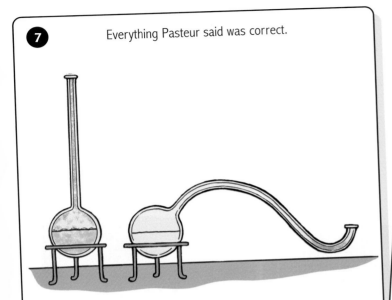

He had proved that germs did not come alive on their own. Germs will only be found in places they are able to reach. They infect things and turn them bad! The theory of 'spontaneous generation' was dead.

8 In 1861, Pasteur published his '**Germ Theory**'. But he had other ideas.

> *If liquid is damaged by germs, then the same can and must happen in men and animals.*

In 1865, he got to test his theory that disease in animals is caused by germs.

9 The French silk industry was being ruined by a disease that was killing their silkworms (the caterpillars that spin silk).

> *I have been called in to solve their problem.*

SILK FACTORY

Through a series of experiments, Pasteur proved that they were dying of a disease called pébrine and it was being spread by a living organism — a germ — in the air!

Pasteur had made a momentous breakthrough. He had proven that germs were all around us ... and some of them could be harmful and cause disease. But Pasteur was a chemist and not a doctor. All of his experiments were carried out on liquids such as beer, milk and wine or silkworms. Many doctors didn't even entertain the thought that germs could damage humans too. They thought it ridiculous that something as small as a germ could harm something as large and advanced as a human.

It ␣␣ a German doctor, Robert Koch, to apply
␣␣ theories to human diseases – and prove
␣␣ s caused most of them.

The importance of Robert Koch

Robert Koch was born in Germany in 1843. As a young man, he became fascinated by Pasteur's 'Germ Theory' and in 1871, his wife bought him a microscope for his birthday. He soon took a particular interest in an especially horrible disease called anthrax. This causes terrible sores on the lungs and can kill humans and animals.

Koch found a way of staining and growing the particular germ he felt was responsible for anthrax in a Petri dish (named after his assistant Julius Petri). He then proved it was this bacterium that caused the disease by injecting mice and making them ill. For the first time, he was able to prove that germs cause disease in humans. As well as anthrax, he was able to identify the germs causing the deadly diseases TB and cholera. In 1905, he was awarded the Nobel Prize for his work.

And what about Pasteur?

Koch's success spurred Pasteur into a flurry of action. By using old or heat-weakened germs, Pasteur developed vaccines for two animal diseases: chicken cholera and anthrax. He went on to develop a vaccination for a particularly revolting animal disease that affects humans too – rabies.

Koch and Pasteur

Between them, Koch and Pasteur encouraged a whole new generation of scientists to dive into the world of deadly disease and search for the germs that caused them. Soon, the germs responsible for typhus, tetanus, typhoid, pneumonia, meningitis, plague, septicaemia and dysentery were identified. And the scientists now had a powerful new weapon to fight infection – vaccines!

Source A ➤ *The 'Father of the Germ Theory', Louis Pasteur. In 1879, Pasteur was investigating chicken cholera, a disease that was crippling the French poultry industry. Pasteur extracted cholera germs from chickens and began trying to make a weak form of it. They had no success. When returning from a holiday, Pasteur's assistant accidentally injected some chickens with an old batch of germs that had been left out, exposed to the air over the holiday. When the same chickens were injected with a new batch of cholera germs, they didn't become ill – the old solution had immunised the chickens against the disease. Pasteur called this method of injecting a weakened form of disease in order to immunise 'vaccination', in honour of Edward Jenner.*

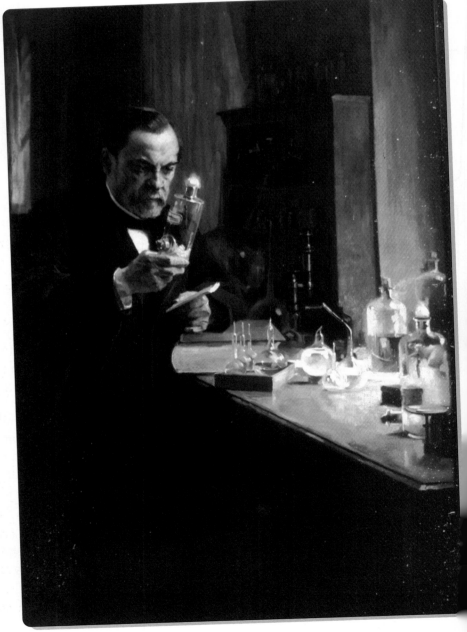

Source B ➤ *Pasteur speaking in a lecture in 1864. He was a great showman who loved doing his experiments in public.*

"So gentlemen, I have taken my drop of water. But it is dead. It is dead because I have kept it from the only thing man cannot produce, from the germs that float in the air, from Life, for Life is a germ and a germ is Life. Never will the theory of spontaneous generation recover from the mortal blow of this simple experiment."

FACT *Germs*

The word 'germ' is a bit of a nickname. 'Germs' are, in reality, living micro-organisms that grow and grow, making a patient worse and worse. Another word for growing is 'germinating' – hence 'germ'.

FACT *France vs Germany*

Frenchman Pasteur and Koch the German were great rivals. This was mainly due to the fact that their countries were great rivals at the time too. During 1870–71, France lost a bitter war to Germany, a war in which Koch served as a doctor in the German army. The defeat made Pasteur hate Germany. The two men used science to compete with each other – and made a series of outstanding advances as a result!

WISE UP WORDS

- miasma   spontaneous generation
  Germ Theory

CLASSIC EXAM QUESTION

1 Explain the theory of spontaneous generation

2 Explain how Pasteur proved this theory wrong

3 How far do you agree with this statement: "Koch's work was more important than Pasteur's."

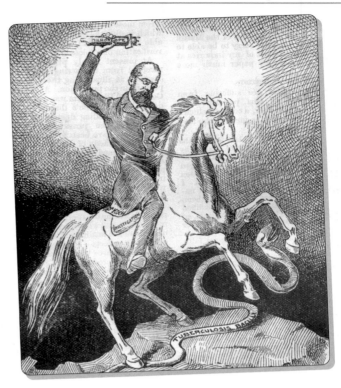

Source C ▲ *A cartoon of Koch from the 1880s. It shows Koch slaying the bacteria responsible for tuberculosis (TB).*

WORK

1 **a** Explain what is meant by the following:
   - the miasma theory
   - the theory of spontaneous generation.
   b Why do you think people believed these theories?

2 In your own words, explain how Pasteur discovered:
   i) the process of pasteurisation;
   ii) that the theory of spontaneous generation was wrong;
   iii) that germs could harm animals.

3 Look at **Source C**.
   a Who is Robert Koch?
   b What is happening in the cartoon?
   c Do you think the cartoonist admired and supported Koch's work or not? Give reasons for your answer.

4 Pasteur once wrote that luck and hard work go together. He said, 'in the fields of observation, chance favours only the mind which is prepared.' Is this true of:
   i) Pasteur's own work?
   ii) Koch's work?
   Explain your answers.

How was public health improved?

Exam Focus

▶ Make sure you know about:
- the state of towns in the early nineteenth century and the dangers this posed to people's health;
- why governments were reluctant to improve public health;
- the reasons why – and how – public health was improved in the late nineteenth century;
- the impact of Chadwick, Snow and Bazalgette.

The health and well-being of ordinary men, women and children (known as 'public health') was in a pretty poor state in 1800. The average age of death for a working man was about 30 – that's right, 30 years of age! In some places, like Liverpool, it was 15! In Manchester, one in every five children died before their first birthday and one in three died before they reached their fifth. The death rate (that is, the number of people in every thousand of the population who die each year) had reached 39 by 1800! In fact, despite improved medical knowledge and understanding, people's health in general may even have been worse in 1800 than the health of people living in earlier centuries. So much for the theory that things always get better!

So why was public health in crisis? What was done to improve it? And what was the state of the nation's health like by 1900?

Disease in the slums

Source A ▾ *Back-to-back housing at Staithes, Yorkshire.*

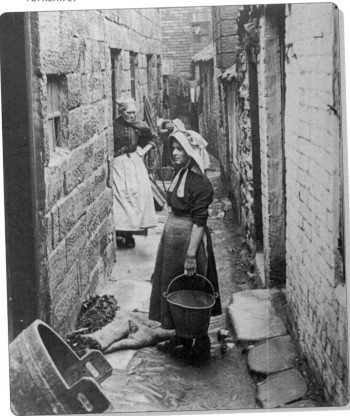

Lots of towns and cities grew very fast in the first 50 years of the 1800s ... and the health of the people living in them grew steadily worse! In 1750, Sheffield, for example, had a population of just 12 000 people. By 1850, the number had risen to over 150 000! People had flocked to Sheffield for one simple reason – to get a job in one of the new factories ... and the promise of the new life that went with it! These new factories, built all over the north and Midlands of England in the early 1800s, needed thousands of workers to operate machinery that made cloth, pottery, iron or steel. And as a single factory alone might employ hundreds of people, rows of houses were built quickly, 'back-to-back', to squeeze as many workers as possible into each street. Almost all the houses were crowded, often with five or more people living in one small room. In 1847, 40 people were found sharing one room in Liverpool.

And none of these houses had toilets either. The best some families could manage was a bucket in the corner of the room that would be emptied now and again, either into the street or stored outside the door until there was enough to sell to a farmer as manure. Occasionally, there was a shared street toilet (a deep hole with a wooden shed over it) but this would be shared by lots of families. Sometimes a water pump provided water, but often the water only came from the local river or pond – and this would be as filthy as the water in the streets.

Sewage trickled down the streets and into nearby rivers – yet most families washed their clothes, their bodies and drank from the same river. It was little wonder that terrible diseases like typhoid, tuberculosis and cholera were common. But no one knew how you *really* caught them – or how you could prevent them. And there were no rubbish collections, no street cleaners or sewers and no fresh running water. Things needed to change … and change fast!

Source B ▾ *From a parliamentary debate.*

"Out of 3000 families in Bury, 773 of them slept three and four in a bed; 209 families had five in a bed; 67 six in a bed and in 15 families, seven slept in one bed … in Liverpool there were 7860 cellars that were dark, damp, small, badly ventilated and dirty. 39 000 people had to live in them."

Source C ▾ *The writer, Charles Reade, describing Sheffield in 1850.*

"Perhaps the most hideous town in creation … sparkling streams enter the town but soon got filthy, full of rubbish, clogged with dirt and bubbling with rotten, foul-smelling gases."

TOP EXAM TIP

Remember that health varied from place to place and from class to class in the 19th century.

Source D ▾ *A plan of back-to-back housing in Nottingham, 1845.*

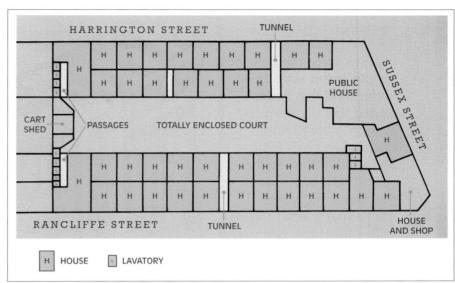

H HOUSE   L LAVATORY

Source E ▾ *Common diseases of the 1800s.*

Disease	Cause	Description
Typhoid	Contaminated water or food.	Spread by poor sanitation or unhygienic conditions. Sewage would get into the water supply that people would drink.
Tuberculosis (TB)	Germs passed in the air through sneezing or coughing.	Spread like 'wild fire' in crowded conditions. Another type of TB was caused by infected cows' milk.
Cholera	Contaminated food or water like typhoid.	Several cholera epidemics swept the country in the early 1800s.

WORK

1 Give as many reasons as you can why it was so easy for disease to spread in large cities in the 1800s.

2 Look at **Source D**.
   a Draw the plan of back-to-back houses.
   b What is missing from these houses that we take for granted today?
   c On your plan, mark which house (or houses) you would least like to live in. Give reasons for your choice.

Here comes cholera!

In filthy, overcrowded cities like Leeds, Liverpool, Bradford and Manchester, diseases spread quickly. But people at this time didn't understand that germs caused their illnesses. Far away in laboratories, doctors like Louis Pasteur had started to make the connection, but down in the streets and slums of Britain, people continued to live their lives and get their filthy water in the same ways as they had always done.

In 1831, a new and frightening disease arrived in Britain – cholera. In this year alone, it killed around 50 000 people. Victims were violently sick and suffered from painful diarrhoea; their skin and nails turned black just before the victim fell into a coma and died. So many people were dying that cemeteries had to be closed because they were too full – bodies had started to poke through the earth's surface, letting off a disgusting stench. One vicar in Bilston, West Midlands, even wrote that 'the coffins could not be made fast enough for the dead'.

What frustrated many was the complete lack of knowledge and understanding of this new killer. There were diseases around that killed more people but cholera was something they hadn't experienced before … and it struck with such devastating speed, killing thousands in a few days. And there was no cure! Naturally then, there was widespread interest in how it was caught, how it spread and how you could prevent it.

Most people at this time believed disease was spread by miasma – an infectious mist given off by rotting animals, rubbish and human waste. This led some towns to clean up their streets (see **Source F**) but the importance of clean water still wasn't understood – and anyway, by 1832, the cholera epidemic had passed and life was getting back to normal. Perhaps cholera would never return!

Source F ▼ *A drawing from the 1830s showing tar barrels being burnt on the streets of Exeter. The smell from the tar was thought to stop the miasma spreading cholera along the street.*

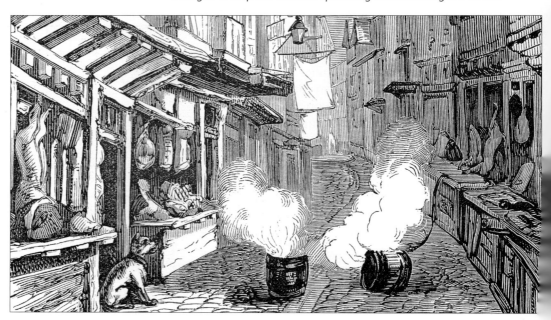

Action at last

After more outbreaks of cholera in 1837 and 1838, the government decided to act. In 1839, they set up an inquiry to find out what living conditions and the health of the poor was like all over Britain. The man in charge was a government official named Edwin Chadwick. Over a two-year period, he sent out doctors to most major towns and cities who filled in questionnaires and interviewed hundreds of people. The *Report on the Sanitary Conditions of the Labouring Population of Great Britain* was published in 1842 (see **Source H**).

Chadwick's report shocked Britain. Over 10 000 free copies were handed out to politicians, journalists, writers and anyone who could change public opinion. Twenty thousand more were sold to the public.

It didn't really matter for now that Chadwick mistakenly believed in the miasma theory. What was important was the fact that the report highlighted the need for cleaner streets and a clean water supply. And the report showed that most people were wrong in thinking that the poor were to blame for bad housing and living conditions. In fact, there was little they could do about it – it was parliament who would have to do something to improve public health.

So what did they do?

Source G ▶ Conclusions of Chadwick's report.

'Disease is caused by bad air and these diseases are common all over the country.'

'A medical officer should be appointed to take charge in each district.'

'People cannot develop clean habits until they have clean water.'

'The poor conditions produce a population that doesn't live long, is always short of money, is brutal and rough.'

'The bad air is caused by rotting animals and vegetables, by damp and filth and by stuffy overcrowded houses. When these things are improved, the death rate goes down.'

'More people are killed by filth and bad ventilation each year than are killed by wars.'

'The poor cost us too much; the rich pay to feed and clothe orphans. Money would be saved if fewer parents died of disease. A healthier workforce would work harder too.'

'We must improve sewers and drains so rubbish is flushed clean away rather than left to rot even more.'

'We must improve drainage, remove rubbish from houses, streets and roads and improve the water supply.'

TOP EXAM TIP

Edwin Chadwick is a great example of the role of an individual as a factor for change.

Source H ▼ Chadwick's report showed that the length of people's lives was greatly affected by where they lived. He told wealthier people who lived in the cities that they would benefit if they paid for improvements. He said they didn't live as long as people in Rutland (a countryside area) because they occasionally caught diseases from people who lived in the slums and delivered goods to their houses or met in the streets. He said that improving the poor areas would improve the health of the rich too!

	Gentlemen	Labourers
Wiltshire	50	33
Liverpool	35	15
Manchester	38	17
Leeds	44	19
Bethnal Green	35	15

WORK

1 Why do you think cholera was one of the most feared diseases of the 1800s?

2 Look at **Source F.** Why are these people burning tar in the streets?

3 Look at **Source G.**
   a Make a list of changes Chadwick wanted to make.
   b What evidence is there that Chadwick believed in the miasma theory?
   c Do you think Chadwick felt sorry for the poor? Explain your answer carefully.

4 Look at **Source H.**
   a Why do you think 'gentlemen' lived longer than 'labourers'?
   b Why do you think people in Wiltshire lived longer than people in Liverpool?

Cholera is back!

Many people paid attention to Chadwick's pleas for improvements. But the government didn't do anything. In the 1800s, many thought politicians had no right to meddle in the private lives of citizens. This attitude was known as **laissez faire**, French words meaning 'leave alone'. It was the job of government to keep law and order, not to keep people clean. And some members of parliament were making vast fortunes from the rent on the slums – tearing them down and rebuilding them would cost them money!

But cholera changed their minds. As news reached Britain of another cholera epidemic sweeping across Europe, the government passed a Public Health Act in 1848 (see **Source J**).

Source I ▼ *The Public Health Act of 1848.*

THE 1848 PUBLIC HEALTH ACT

- A NATIONAL BOARD OF HEALTH IS TO BE CREATED WITH THE POWER TO SET UP LOCAL HEALTH BOARDS [COMMITTEES THAT TRY TO IMPROVE DRAINAGE, SEWERS, RUBBISH COLLECTIONS, BUILD 'PUBLIC TOILETS', WATER SUPPLIES AND SO ON] WHERE THERE IS A HIGH DEATH RATE.

- LOCAL BOARDS OF HEALTH HAVE POWERS TO:
  - MAKE SURE NEW HOUSES ARE BUILT WITH DRAINS AND TOILETS
  - CHARGE A LOCAL RATE (TAX) TO PAY FOR IMPROVEMENTS
  - APPOINT MEDICAL OFFICERS WHO CAN 'INSPECT NUISANCES'

The Act gave local town councils the power to spend money on cleaning up their towns if they wanted to. Some towns, like Liverpool and Birmingham, made huge improvements, but many others didn't bother to do anything. Only 103 towns had set up their own Boards of Health by 1853.

Meanwhile, the plague of cholera continued. In 1848, 60 000 people died, followed by 20 000 in 1854. During the 1854 epidemic, a doctor named John Snow made a major breakthrough in proving there was a link between cholera and water supply. Perhaps the breakthrough would lead the government to do even more about public health!

Discovering the cause of cholera

Doctor John Snow was a famous surgeon who worked in Broad Street, Soho, London. In 1854, over 700 people living in this street, or nearby streets, died of cholera within ten days. Snow began to investigate.

Through meticulous research, Snow found that all victims in this small area got their water from the Broad Street water pump. Those who didn't die seemed to be getting their water from other places. Snow asked permission to remove the handle of the water pump so people were forced to use another. There were no more deaths in the street! Snow investigated further and found that a street toilet, only one metre from the pump, had a cracked lining that allowed polluted water to trickle into the drinking water. Snow had proved that cholera was not carried through the air like a poisonous gas or an infectious mist (so called 'miasma'); instead it was caught through contagion – by coming into direct contact with a cholera sufferer or in this case, drinking some water contaminated by a victim's diarrhoea.

The discovery that cholera was a water-borne disease was a remarkable achievement. Pasteur didn't publish his Germ Theory until 1860, which would have helped to explain the results Snow had recorded.

So the government now had a growing batch of evidence about the state of the nation's health within the dirty, overcrowded towns. They even had medical evidence that made a link between cholera and water supply. So what did the government do about it? Not a lot! But more and more politicians were being persuaded that a countrywide clean up was needed … and the Great Stink finally forced them into action.

TOP EXAM TIP

*Dr Snow used scientific observation to show **how** cholera spread – but he didn't know **why** it spread. You need to understand the difference.*

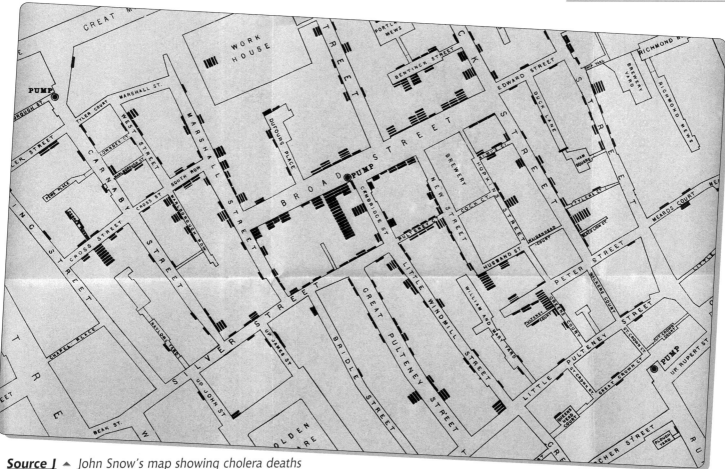

Source J ▲ *John Snow's map showing cholera deaths (shown as black blocks) between 19 August and 30 September, 1854.*

Source K ◄ *A cartoon called* The Silent Highway Man, *from Punch magazine, 10 July 1858. Do you think this cartoonist agrees or disagrees with Snow?*

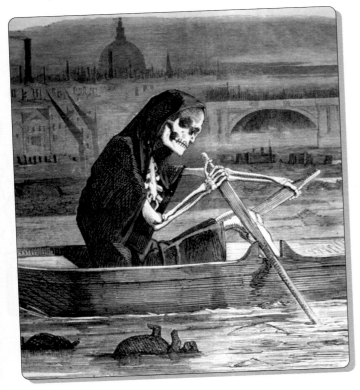

WORK

1 **a** What is meant by the term 'laissez faire'?

   b Why do you think so many politicians believed in 'laissez faire'?

2 **a** List some of the things that Local Boards of Health could do.

   b Why do you think public toilets were far more important in the nineteenth century than they are today?

   c What were the limitations of the First Public Health Act of 1848?

3 Imagine you are Doctor John Snow. Write a letter to the National Board of Health explaining:

   i) how you think cholera is spread (you will need to summarise your evidence);

   ii) what you think should be done about it.

The Great Stink

In the summer of 1858, a heat wave caused the filthy River Thames to smell worse than ever. For years, human sewage, dead animals, household rubbish, horse dung, slaughterhouse waste and chemicals from factories had been dumped in the River – and now the heat had made the stench intolerable. The smell was so bad that the politicians in the Houses of Parliament (right next to the River) demanded to meet somewhere else. Some even started to call London 'the Great Stink'. So what were the MPs going to do about it? Finally, it seems that the smell inspired them into action!

The stench from the Thames and Snow's new evidence about cholera caused such alarm that MPs turned to a man they hoped could save their city. His name was Joseph Bazalgette.

Three years earlier, he had been asked to draw up plans for a network of underground tunnels – or sewers – to collect all the waste from nearly one million London houses before it had a chance to flow into the Thames. Powerful pumps, the largest ever made, would then push all the sewage along the tunnels and out towards the sea. Now the MPs wanted London's streets free of sewage … quickly. Bazalgette was given £3 million (about £1 billion today) and told to start immediately (see **Source N**).

▼ *MPs fleeing the smell!*

Using 318 million bricks, he built 83 miles of sewers, removing 420 million gallons of sewage a day. They were finished in 1866 – and when fully operational, cholera never retuned to London. Soon, parliament went into a flurry of action (see **Source O**).

Source L ▼ *Acts to make places healthier.*

MAKING TOWNS HEALTHIER

1866 Sanitary Act – Towns must install a proper water supply and sewage disposal system at once. Inspectors will check this has been done.

1875 Housing Act – Councils have the power to pull down the worst houses in the worst areas and build better homes.

1875 Public Health Act – Local councils must keep the pavements lit, paved and cleaned. Sewers must be clean and rubbish cleared from the streets. They may increase taxes to pay for this.

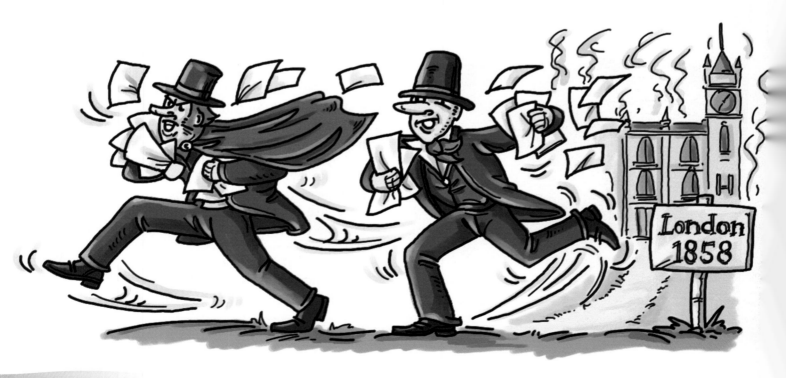

Source M ▾ *A Punch cartoon commenting on the state of the Thames in 1858.*

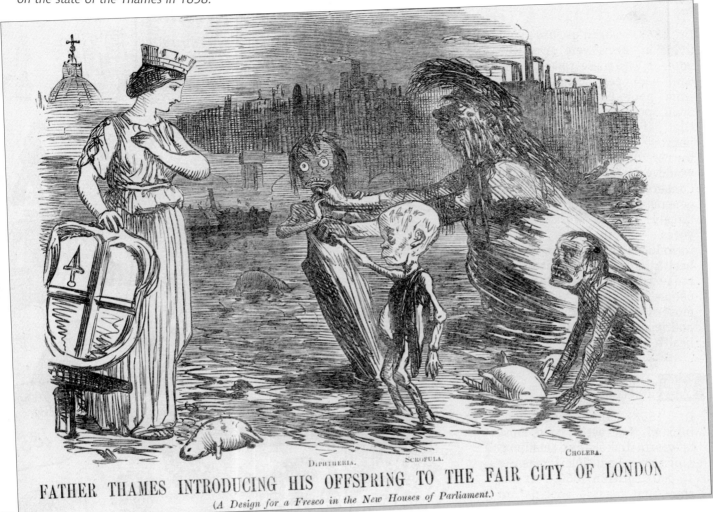

DIPHTHERIA. SCROFULA. CHOLERA.

FATHER THAMES INTRODUCING HIS OFFSPRING TO THE FAIR CITY OF LONDON

(A Design for a Fresco in the New Houses of Parliament.)

Source N ◂ *Many of Bazalgette's sewers are still used below London's streets today. Bazalgette is pictured here, above the sewers, on the right.*

WORK

1 **a** Why was London known as the 'Great Stink' in 1858?

 b Cholera never returned to London after Bazalgette's sewers were fully operational. Have Londoners got just Bazalgette to thank for this? Explain your answer.

2 Look at **Source M**. What is the message of this cartoon?

FACT *The death of laissez faire*

In 1867, working-class men living in towns were given the vote. It was these same people who had been suffering most from poor living conditions. Soon, political parties realised that if they promised to improve conditions in the towns, the people living there would vote for them. When the Conservative Party won the general election in 1874, it was largely due to working-class votes. Soon after, they introduced many new public health reforms. Many historians today think that working-class people getting the vote is the most important reason why politicians began to improve the health of the nation.

FACT *Injection action*

In 1853, the government insisted that every baby must be vaccinated against smallpox, a disease responsible for nearly 10 000 deaths in 1850. This was the first mass vaccination programme of its kind and deaths from smallpox soon dropped dramatically.

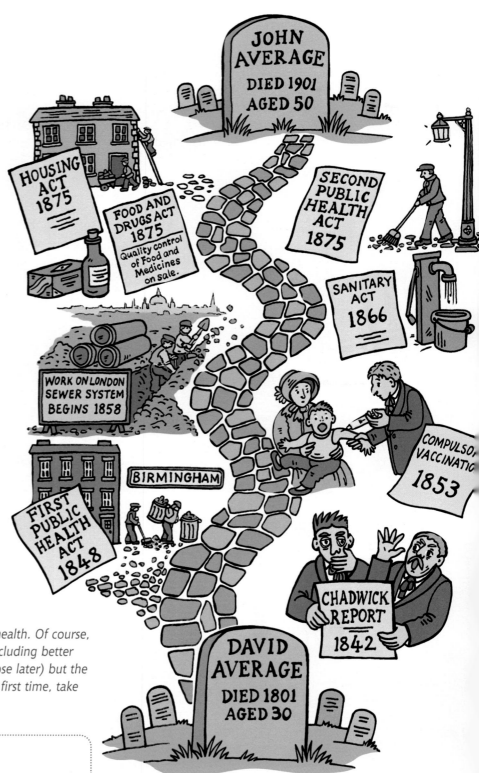

Source O ▸ *The road to improved public health. Of course, other measures improved life expectancy, including better nursing and surgery techniques (more of those later) but the nineteenth century saw government, for the first time, take some responsibility for public health.*

FACT *Getting better?*

The death rate fell from about 39 in 1800 to 18 in 1900. The average age of death rose from 30 to 50 and the total population of the country rose from about ten million in 1801 to 38 million in 1901. So the population increased nearly four times – mainly because people were living longer.

CLASSIC EXAM QUESTION

How and why had public health improved in towns by the end of the 19th century?

But what about the kids?

The health of children in the nineteenth century is a very sad story. Whilst the death rate for adults dropped sharply, the rate for children actually increased to the shocking figure of 142 per 1000 in 1899. In some areas, it was much worse. In York, for example, it was 250 per 1000 – that meant *one quarter* of their children died before their first birthday. Why?

Many of the babies that survived childhood were deformed and sickly. The sorry state of young people was confirmed in 1899 when a big army recruiting campaign took place. It was found that 40 out of every 100 young men who volunteered were 'unfit for service' – even for the army's relatively low standards. Clearly, the improvement in children's health is one of the greatest achievements of the twentieth century, not the nineteenth!

WISE UP WORD
- Laissez faire

Doctors cost money
There was no free medical treatment so families still used their own homemade medicines. The expense of calling a doctor was often put off until it was too late.

Overcrowding
With families of ten or more sharing two or three rooms, infectious diseases spread very quickly – and small children easily pick up infection.

Wrong food
Lack of education meant that babies were often given too little, too much or the wrong food. Bread and meat were given to babies at a very young age and their stomachs couldn't cope.

Why did the health of children decline?

Drugs
Tired parents often 'doped' their babies because they couldn't cope with screaming infants who were hungry or ill. Opium could be bought in penny bottles from a chemist. Sometimes the babies never woke up.

Neglect
In a period of great darkness, many babies just weren't looked after. The money that could have been spent on children was sometimes spent on beer and gin instead.

Filthy housing
Ordinary men and women didn't know the value of keeping a clean house. In the 1880s, over 12 000 babies a year died of diarrhoea caused mainly by dirt.

WORK

1 a Summarise the reasons why the health of children didn't improve as much as adults in the nineteenth century.

   b Choose three factors that you think would be most difficult to solve. Explain your choices.

2 Design a poster that explains the improvements made in public health in the nineteenth century. Your poster should include information on:

- common killer diseases of the 1800s and how some were combated;
- death rates, life expectancy and so on, 1800–1900;
- influential men like Chadwick, Snow, Bazalgette;
- government action;
- the health of children 1800–1900.

NOTE: Aim your poster at someone who has never studied health and medicine at GCSE before. Include no more than 250 words on your poster.

Hospitals from hell?

Exam Focus

▸ For your exam, you will need to know how the problems of pain and infectiion during and after surgery were overcome during the nineteenth century.

Look at **Source A**. It is a painting from 1750. The patient is in absolute agony. Look at his face; he is being held down whilst surgeons cut off his leg. The poor man won't have been given any painkilling drugs – he is completely awake when the surgeon starts to slice into his skin and saw through his thighbone. It is highly unlikely that the medical equipment being used has ever been washed either. It will be stained with the dry blood and pus from a previous patient. One well-known surgeon used to sharpen his knives on the sole of his boot before using them, and you know how filthy the streets were! What do you think the patient's chances of survival were? Why were conditions so bad? And why have they improved so much since then?

In 1750, a patient in a British hospital had two major enemies. One was the pain during the operation; the other was infection afterwards. Either could kill you!

Source A ▾ *We can't even begin to imagine what sort of pain this patient was in!*

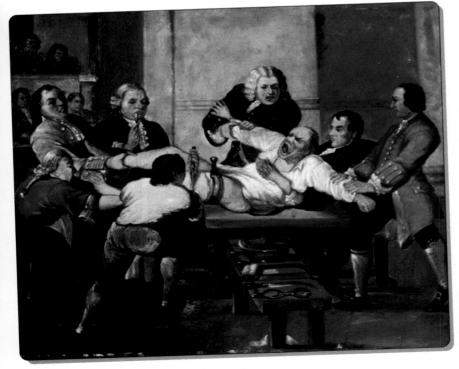

Only when these two obstacles were dealt with would it be possible to make any real medical progress. In the nineteenth century, doctors started to find the solutions to these problems … and changed the way the sick were cared for forever!

For hundreds of years, doctors and surgeons had tried to reduce a patient's pain during surgery. Getting them drunk or hitting them over the head were two of the most common methods. But in 1846, an American dentist called William Moston tried out a new idea. He put his patients to sleep for a short period of time using a gas called **ether**. It worked! The patient felt no pain during the operation, woke up 20 minutes later and went home. Anaesthetics (based on the word 'ether') were born and the idea soon caught on amongst London's surgeons after a doctor named J R Liston amputated a man's diseased leg. When the patient woke up after an hour-long operation, he asked, 'When are you going to start?'! However, ether irritated patients' eyes and made them cough and vomit during operations.

In 1847, a Scottish doctor called James Simpson tried using a new and untested gas – **chloroform** – as an alternative to ether.

He had discovered its 'knock-out' properties in quite an amusing way (see **Source B**). He used it mainly to relieve women's labour pains during childbirth and noted that it had fewer of the nasty side effects of ether.

But as we have seen with most new medical discoveries, the first reaction of most surgeons was intense criticism and opposition. Some argued that the long-term side effects were unknown whilst others put forward their arguments on religious grounds. They said that it was unnatural to ease a woman's pain during childbirth, for example, as 'pain may be considered as a blessing of the Gospel'. Simpson's cause wasn't helped when, in 1848, a patient named Hannah Greener died after being given chloroform during an operation to remove her toenail!

So the arguments surrounding the use of anaesthetics (in particular, chloroform) continued for years. Sometimes Simpson himself met with doctors and put up a spirited defence of their use (see **Source C**). However, the final breakthrough in their acceptance came from none other than Queen Victoria herself. In 1857, she used chloroform during the delivery of her eighth baby. With the Queen's support, it wasn't long before the use of anaesthetics became common in surgical practice.

Source B ➤ *Simpson and two other doctor friends experimented with different chemicals in order to find one that could be used as an anaesthetic. When Simpson poured some chloroform into a glass on the table, he and his friends were 'under the table in a minute, much to my wife's alarm'.*

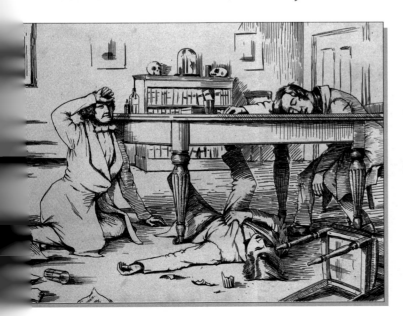

Source C ➤ *James Simpson speaking at a meeting in 1847.*

"Before the sixteenth century, surgeons had no way of stemming the flow of blood after amputation of a limb other than by scorching with a red hot iron or boiling pitch. The great suggestion of Ambroise Paré to shut up the bleeding vessels by tying them was a vast improvement. It saved the sufferings of the patients while adding to their safety. But the practice was new and, like all innovations in medical practice, it was at first and for long, bitterly decried ... attacked ... suppressed.

We look back with sorrow on the opponents of Paré. Our successors in years to come will look back with similar feelings. They will marvel at the idea of humane men confessing that they prefer operating on their patients in a waking instead of an anaesthetic state and that the fearful agonies that they inflict should be endured quietly. All pain is destructive and even fatal in its effects."

The use of anaesthetics was a great step forward, but it didn't stop people dying from infections after operations. Today, we take it for granted that our hospitals and operating theatres are very, very clean, but in the early 1800s, it was a very different story. Hospitals were dirty places, where patients were all herded together, whether they had a highly contagious fever or a broken arm. The operating theatres were no better. The only thing that was ever cleaned out was the sand box from under the operating table, which was used to catch the patients' blood during surgery. The cockroaches in St Thomas' Hospital were said to be the biggest in London. They fed on dried blood and dead skin. Doctors and surgeons didn't understand the need for cleanliness because they didn't know that germs caused disease. It would take a few more famous men to solve this problem!

FACT *Record breaker*

In the 1840s, a famous London surgeon named Robert Liston held the world record for **amputating** a leg – two and a half minutes. Unfortunately, he worked so fast that he accidentally cut off the patient's testicles! Also, he once cut off his assistant's fingers during another operation and a spectator dropped dead with fright.

By the 1850s then, surgeons were performing much better operations. As their patients were unconscious due to the anaesthetic, surgeons could take their time and work carefully – and they didn't run the risk of their patient dying of shock. At Leeds Hospital, for example, the number of tricky operations on the stomach, intestines and ovaries rose from 15 a year to over 100. However, patients continued to die of blood poisoning and nasty infections. After all, the doctors were operating on old wooden tables, in dirty rooms, in their ordinary clothes, using unwashed instruments that had been used on several other patients that day. Many doctors just didn't realise the danger of it (see **Source D**)!

Source D ▼ *'Sepsis' is the Greek word for 'rotten'. The farmer's wound had gone rotten and he had died from blood poisoning. In fact, the number of patients dying after operations in the 1850s was astonishing – as many as six out of ten!*

> "A strong, young farmer came in to the hospital and told the surgeon that his girlfriend had made comments about his nose — it was too much to one side; could it be straightened? He had heard of the wonderful things that were done in London hospitals. He was admitted; the septum [bone between the nostrils] was straightened and in five days he was dead. He died of hospital sepsis."

How did the Germ Theory affect surgery?

In 1861, Louis Pasteur published his Germ Theory. In it, he said he had proved that tiny creatures, or germs, make milk, beer and wine go bad. These germs also caused disease in silkworms. He went on to suggest that germs also caused human diseases. This was a major breakthrough and finally put to an end many of the old ideas about the causes of disease such as bad air (miasma) and the theory of the four humours!

Pasteur went on to say that many of these germs could be killed by heat – and proved this in his laboratory. He even offered some advice to surgeons (see **Source E**).

Source E ▼ *Louis Pasteur.*

> "If I were a surgeon, impressed as I am with the dangers to which the patient is exposed to microbes [germs] present over the surface of all objects, particularly in hospitals, not only would I use none but perfectly clean instruments, but after having cleansed my hands with the greatest care, and subjected them to a rapid flaming … I would use only lint, bandages and sponges previously exposed to a temperature of 130°C to 150°C."

Source F ▼ *Antiseptic in action. An operation using Lister's carbolic acid spray. Note the doctor on the left is putting the patient 'to sleep' with the anaesthetic.*

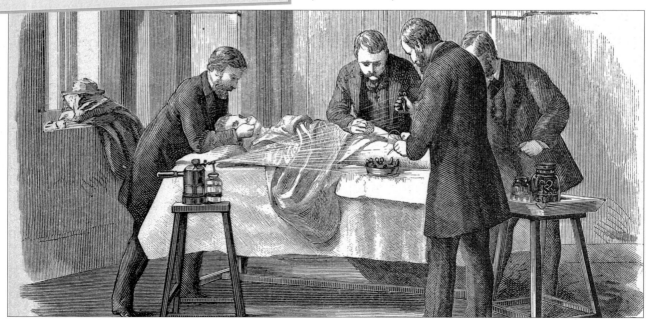

In 1867, an English surgeon, Joseph Lister, applied Pasteur's theories to his work at the newly opened Glasgow Royal Infirmary. He thought that it might be germs that caused so many of his patients to die from sepsis. Surely, he believed, if the germs were killed with antiseptic ('anti' means against), then more of his patients would survive. Lister chose carbolic acid as his antiseptic. Using a pump, a bit like an aerosol can, he sprayed anything that might possibly come into contact with the wound. Spray everything, he hoped, and all the germs would die. He was right! His patients didn't get any infection and antiseptics were born (see **Source F**).

Source G ▼ *As you might expect, Lister's new methods met with opposition. Carbolic acid irritated the surgeon's hands and the patient's flesh. And it made everything smell! However, the following figures, from Lister's own records, allow the success of carbolic acid to speak for itself.*

	Total amputations	Died	% who died
1864–1866 (without antiseptics)	35	16	46%
1867–1870 (with antiseptics)	40	6	15%

Soon doctors and surgeons all over the country were trying antiseptic sprays and other cleaner ways to work. Hospitals waged a war against germs. Walls were scrubbed clean, floors were swept and equipment was **sterilised**. Surgeons started to wear rubber gloves, surgical gowns and facemasks during operations (see **Source H**).

The results of these measures were plain to see. Hospitals started to cure more people than they killed. Astonishingly, figures from Newcastle Infirmary, published in 1878, show that before antiseptics were introduced, six out of ten people died after operations. After antiseptics, only one out of every ten died!

And soon after, surgeons attempted more and more ambitious operations. The first successful appendix operation was performed in 1883 and the first heart operation took place in 1896 (to repair a stab wound).

WISE UP WORDS

• ether   chloroform   amputation   sterilised

Source H ▼ *An operation in 1900. Look for all the different ways in which this surgeon tries to keep a cleaner operating room.*

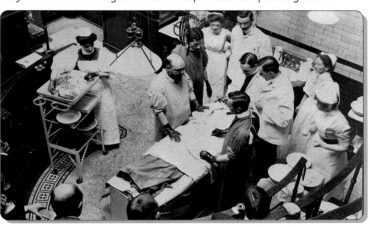

WORK

1 Look at **Source A**.
  a Write a brief description of the scene in this source. Use no more than 100 words.
  b Make a list of things in **Source A** that would not happen during surgery today.

2 a What is an anaesthetic?
  b Why did chloroform become the most popular form of anaesthetics?
  c How did Queen Victoria help anaesthetics to be accepted?
  d How did surgery change when anaesthetics were introduced?

3 Look at **Sources E** and **F**.
  a Explain what is meant by the term 'antiseptic'.
  b How was Lister's work linked to Pasteur's Germ Theory?

4 Look at **Sources A** and **H**.
  a Draw two spider diagrams, each describing the main features of an operation in 1750 and 1900.
  b Write a paragraph comparing how the two operations have changed.
  c Look at your 1900 diagram and think about an operation in a modern hospital today. Circle the things that have changed since 1900 in one colour and underline the things that still happen today during an operation in another.

CLASSIC EXAM QUESTION

1 Explain some of the objections people had to using anaesthetics

2 How far had problems in surgery been overcome by the end of the 19th century?

Enough about history, what about her story?

Topic Focus

▸ Make sure you know about:
- the difficulties faced by women who wished to go into the medical profession during the nineteenth century;
- the importance of Elizabeth Garrett.

What prevented women from being doctors?

There had been women doctors in the Ancient World but not in the Middle Ages. During Henry V's reign, a law was passed preventing women from practising medicine. Their role was restricted to village healers and midwives or local wise women who had a good knowledge of herbal treatments passed down through generations. However, if any treatment made a patient worse, these women were sometimes accused of being witches!

Surprisingly, there were a few women surgeons in the 1600s who had probably learned their trade by following around their surgeon fathers or brothers. But by 1700, women surgeons had all but disappeared too. It was now compulsory to have a university degree to practise medicine – and women weren't allowed to go to university!

In the 1700s, even the traditional female role of a midwife was under threat. It became fashionable, especially amongst richer families, to have a male doctor at the birth of any children. And as forceps (special instruments used to deliver babies) became more common, men were the only people trained to use them – as they had been the ones permitted to attend university!

Getting qualified

In 1815, doctors and surgeons began to take examinations for their certificates. Hospitals too started to open more schools for training doctors. In 1858, the government introduced the General Medical Act which required all qualified doctors, surgeons and apothecaries (chemists) to put their names on the General Medical Register. If you were not on the list, you were not permitted to practise medicine in any way. In 1858, there was one woman on the list – Elizabeth Blackwell.

The two Elizabeths

Elizabeth Blackwell had qualified as a doctor in 1849 in America, a country that had a more liberal attitude to women attending their universities. Then she came to England to work – and because she was qualified, the General Medical Council had to put her name on their register. In 1859, she met Elizabeth Garrett in London, a young English woman who was determined to follow Blackwell's example.

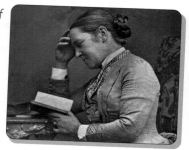

Source A ▸ *A photograph of Elizabeth Garrett. In 1862, she wrote her father a letter saying, 'I think I must act as a pioneer and spend the best years of my life working so that others will reap the benefits.'*

The Elizabeth Garrett story

Elizabeth Garrett's difficulty in gaining status as a doctor was down to the fact that she just couldn't get on any of the courses at medical school. She was turned down by the universities of St Andrew's and Edinburgh because she was a woman. Instead, she found men who would tutor her privately.

In 1865, she managed to pass the Apothecaries' (chemists') examination but they refused to give her a licence to practise. So she sued them – and won – but the Apothecaries' Society said they wouldn't pass any other students who had studied privately. So the door was slammed firmly shut for any more female chemists!

After gaining her Apothecary licence, Garrett was even more determined than ever to become a doctor. She achieved this status in 1869, after studying abroad in Paris. She passed her exams with the highest possible grades.

When Doctor Elizabeth Garrett returned to England, she was placed on the General Medical Register.

So how important was Elizabeth Garrett?

There is no doubt that Elizabeth Garrett was a remarkable woman. She showed great determination to achieve her goals despite the obstacles put in her way. And she certainly paved the way for other women to follow in her footsteps. By seeking qualifications abroad, women like Frances Elizabeth Hoggon (1870), Elizabeth Walker (1872) and Louise Atkins (1872) also became some of Britain's first female doctors.

But there were other characters who contributed to the rise of the female doctor. Sophia Jex-Blake, for example, founded a medical school for women in London in 1874. With 23 students in the first year, enrolments climbed steadily, especially after a university recognised the degrees handed out by Jex-Blake's school.

Recognition at last

During the 1870s, there were many debates in parliament about the case for women's rights in medicine. Finally, in 1876, parliament passed a law that said that women should not be restricted from gaining medical qualifications 'on the grounds of their sex'. In 1881, there were over 25 qualified women doctors on the Medical Register – by 1901, there were 212.

Source C ▾ *Arthur Roebuck, a Liberal MP, speaking in the House of Commons, 3 March 1875.*

"You may talk for a month; you may bring great law to bear upon this question; you may quote names great in history, arts and science. But you cannot rub out the stain which will be on this House if it refuses to do justice for women … and prevents them from using their intellect … in a fair, honest and upright manner for their own good."

Source D ▾ *The number of doctors in the population, according to the population census.*

	Total population	Number of doctors
1841	16 000 000	15 800
1871	23 000 000	14 600

Source E ▾ *Enrolments at the London School of Medicine for Women.*

Year	Number	Year	Number	Year	Number
1875	23	1887	77	1889	91
1892	133	1896	159	1903	318
1917	441				

WORK

1 Explain why it was nearly impossible for women to become doctors in the early 1800s.

2 Look at **Source B**.
   a According to the cartoon, why has the man called out the doctor?
   b What did this show about the attitude of some people to female doctors?

3 Use **Sources A**, **C** and **E** to explain why women were eventually allowed to become doctors.

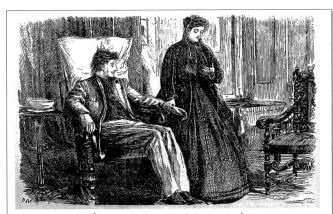

'Who is this interesting invalid?'
It is young Reginald, who has succeeded in catching a bad cold in order that he might send for Doctor Arabella!

◂ **Source B** *A Punch cartoon from 1865 showing the expected effect of women doctors.*

How did Florence Nightingale change nursing?

Topic Focus

▸ These six pages will help you to understand:
- the impact of Florence Nightingale on nursing;
- how nursing became a more respected profession.

Look at **Source A**. It is the back of an old £10 note. The woman pictured on the note is a nurse called Florence Nightingale and her image appeared on £10 notes for seven years between 1975 and 1992. She was the first woman, apart from the Queen, to appear on British banknotes.

Having your image on the back of a bank note is a great honour that is generally reserved for some of Britain's great thinkers, inventors, scientists and composers.

So how did a nurse manage to get her picture on one of Britain's bank notes? What exactly did she do? And how did she change nursing forever?

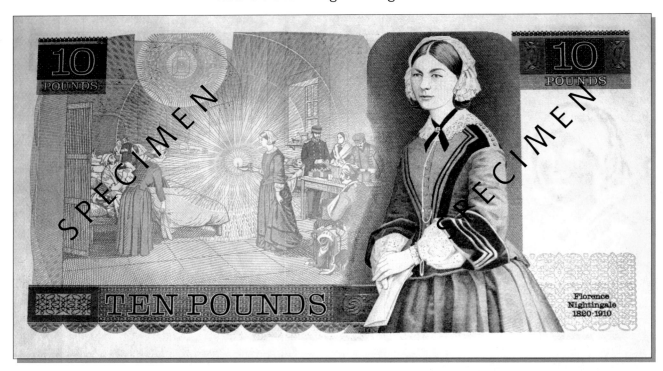

Source A ▲ *The £10 note on which Florence Nightingale appeared. The background image shows a hospital in the Crimea in which Florence Nightingale had made some changes.*

Hospitals in Britain began in various ways. Some, like St Bartholomew's and St Thomas' in London, were started by the Church in the Middle Ages. The Church also started asylums for people with mental illnesses or diseases like leprosy. Local authorities took over some of these places, closing some … and neglecting most of the others. Those that had managed to stay open by the 1700s were filthy places that reminded many of prison!

In the eighteenth century, 'voluntary hospitals' opened in cities all over Britain. These were paid for and used by people who paid a subscription every year. But the poor could not afford the yearly fees so some hospitals were founded that admitted only the very poor – but these places were hotbeds of infection. The rich didn't go near them of course, and conditions were so bad that one historian described the front entrance to one of them as a 'gateway to death'!

The nurses who worked in these places had a bad reputation too. Most of them were untrained – and for many, part of their wages was paid in gin. But by the second half of the 1900s, there had been a transformation in nursing. The person most commonly associated with these changes is Florence Nightingale. Now study carefully her story and the sources that accompany it.

1 Florence Nightingale was born into a wealthy family in 1820.

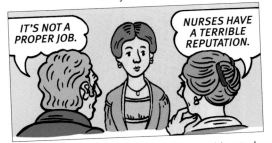

When she told her parents that God wanted her to be a nurse and care for the sick, they were horrified.

2 In 1850, she went to train as a nurse in Germany for three months.

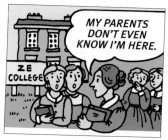

Back in Britain, she got a job running a hospital for rich women — but she wasn't happy doing that.

3 In 1854, war broke out between Britain and Russia in the Crimea.

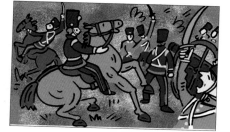

Around 100 000 British soldiers were killed or wounded — but many more fell ill through typhus and other diseases.

4 Reports got back to Britain about the dreadful conditions in the army hospitals.

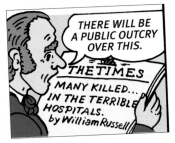

The man in charge of the army knew Florence — and asked her to take control of nursing the troops at the main army hospital in Scutari.

5 Florence took a group of 38 nurses with her to the war zone. She was horrified at the conditions.

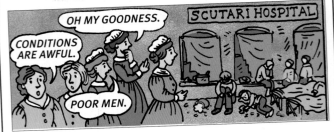

There were no toilet facilities, no cleaning basins, soap, mops, towels or cleaning materials.

6 Florence wrote home to the British government straightaway.

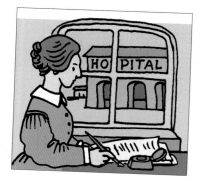

As well as describing conditions, she ordered all sorts of cleaning materials. She even offered to pay for some herself.

7 Florence and her nurses cleaned the hospital from top to bottom — she also hired 200 builders to rebuild part of a ward.

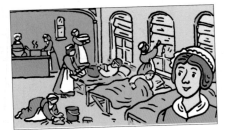

Some of the doctors objected to a nurse telling them how to run their hospital but Florence persisted. She and her nurses removed wheelbarrows full of rubbish.

8 Within six months, she reduced the death rate in the hospital from 40% to 2%.

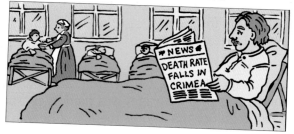

Even the doctors must have been impressed with the increased survival rate amongst the wounded soldiers.

9 Newspapers back in Britain called her the 'Lady with the Lamp' because it was claimed that she walked around at night making sure the soldiers were OK.

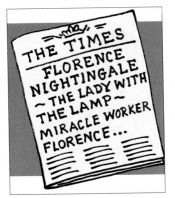

After two years, she returned to Britain as a national hero — but she was very ill!

10 Florence felt that if she could improve hospitals abroad, she could do it in Britain. She immediately wrote a 800-page report to the government telling them how to improve things.

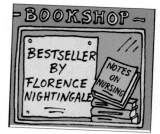

In 1860, her new book, *Notes on Nursing*, became a bestseller. She even visited Queen Victoria to tell her about her experiences.

11 Florence raised £44 000 to set up Britain's first nurse training school at St Thomas' Hospital.

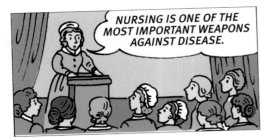

NURSING IS ONE OF THE MOST IMPORTANT WEAPONS AGAINST DISEASE.

She aimed to turn nursing into a respectable profession that could produce well-trained people to go into hospitals and take control of nursing away from men.

12 In 1863, Florence published *Notes on Hospitals*, which introduced new ideas about the design of hospitals.

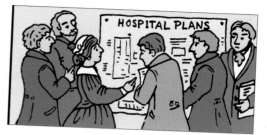

She believed in open, spacious, well-ventilated hospitals because she (mistakenly) thought that stale air spread disease. Countries from all over the world consulted her about hospital design.

Source C ▼ *The wounded in a hospital in the Crimea before Florence Nightingale's arrival.*

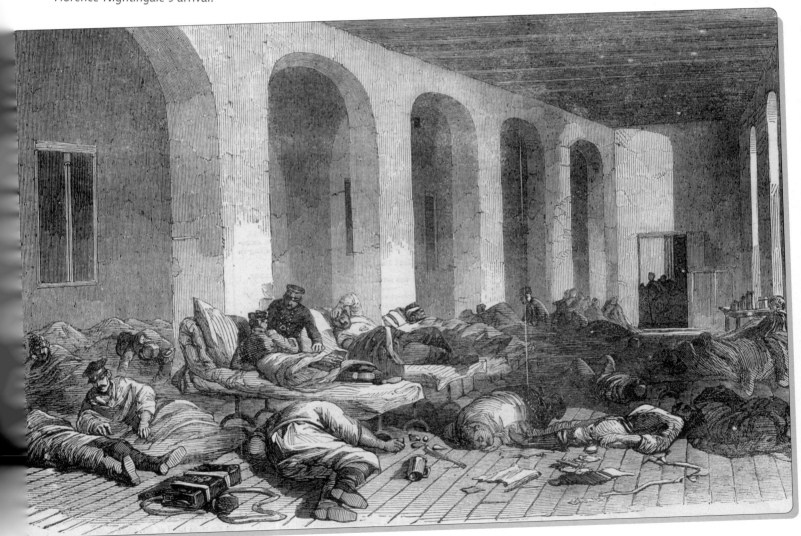

Source D ▼ *One of Nightingale's first letters back to Britain, 25 November 1854.*

"It appears that in these hospitals, the washing of linen and of the men are considered a minor detail. No washing has been performed for the men or the bed — except by ourselves. When we came here, there was neither basin, towel, nor soap in the wards. The consequences of this are Fever, Cholera, Gangrene, Lice, Bugs, Fleas."

Source E ▼ *When student nurses applied for a place at one of Nightingale's schools of nursing, this was printed on the back of the application form.*

DUTIES OF PROBATIONER

YOU ARE REQUIRED TO BE SOBER, HONEST, PUNCTUAL, QUIET AND CLEAN AND NEAT. YOU ARE EXPECTED TO BECOME SKILFUL:

1 IN THE DRESSING OF BLISTERS, BURNS, SORES, WOUNDS AND IN MINOR DRESSINGS.

2 IN THE APPLICATION OF LEECHES.

3 IN THE MANAGEMENT OF HELPLESS PATIENTS, I.E. MOVING, CHANGING, PERSONAL CLEANLINESS OF, FEEDING, AND PREVENTING AND DRESSING BEDSORES.

4 IN BANDAGING AND MAKING BANDAGES.

5 YOU ARE REQUIRED TO ATTEND AT OPERATIONS.

6 TO UNDERSTAND VENTILATION, KEEPING THE WARD FRESH; TO OBSERVE CLEANLINESS IN ALL UTENSILS.

7 TO MAKE OBSERVATIONS OF THE SICK: THE PULSE, APPETITE, BREATHING, STATE OF WOUNDS, EFFECT OF DIET AND MEDICINES.

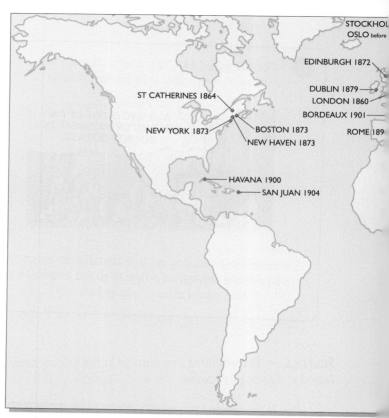

Source F ▲ *A map to show the spread of the Nightingale system of nursing education. The dates show approximately the year of the first nursing school in each country.*

Source G ▼ *Charles E Rosenberg,* Explaining Epidemics and Other Studies in the History of Medicine, *1992.*

"[She was] one of the few individuals who exerted a peculiar and indispensable influence on that history … Her two most widely read books, *Notes on Nursing* and *Notes on Hospitals*, had an extraordinary success in the second half of the century; it would be hard to overestimate her influence in the shaping of modern nursing and the reordering of hospitals."

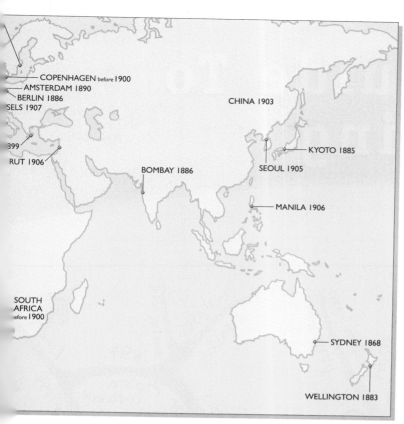

COPENHAGEN before 1900
AMSTERDAM 1890
BERLIN 1886
SELS 1907
399
RUT 1906
CHINA 1903
KYOTO 1885
BOMBAY 1886
SEOUL 1905
MANILA 1906
SOUTH AFRICA before 1900
SYDNEY 1868
WELLINGTON 1883

Source H ▼ *From* Health and Medicine, 1750–1900 *by John Robottom.*

"As they moved to new jobs, usually chosen for them by Florence Nightingale, the lady pupils spread nurse training from St Thomas' to other hospitals. When they chose a 'Nightingale lady' as matron instead of an ex-housekeeper or a respectable widow with no qualifications as matron, hospitals were taking an important decision. They were deciding to treat their nurses as part of the medical team, not as servants."

FACT *Forgotten hero?*

Mary Seacole was another nurse who made her mark during the Crimean War. Born in Jamaica in 1805, she arrived in Britain in 1854 and asked to go out to the Crimea to help British troops. After waiting weeks without getting an interview, she paid to go out herself. When she arrived, she set up a 'British Hotel' where she provided soldiers with a bed for the night and nourishing hot food. On occasions, she went out on to the battlefields to treat wounded men – from both sides of the conflict. As you might expect, she soon won the respect of the troops!

WORK

1 Look at the background picture in **Source A** and **Source C**.

  a What are the main differences between these two scenes?

  b What was Florence Nightingale hoping to achieve by making these changes?

2 Look at **Sources B** and **E**.

  a What image of nurses does **Source B** give?

  b In what ways did Florence Nightingale try to change this image?

3 The portrait in **Source A** is to be used to illustrate an encyclopaedia entry for Florence Nightingale. Write the text for the entry to go with it. Make sure you explain:
  • who she was
  • how she changed nursing
  • why her work was important.

NOTE: your editor has said you can use no more than 50 words!

4 Why do you think Florence Nightingale is best known as the 'Lady with the Lamp' rather than the lady who reorganised nursing?

CLASSIC EXAM QUESTION

  a How similar was the work of Florence Nightingale and Mary Seacole in the Crimea?

  b Explain how the miasma theory influenced Nightingale's work and ideas about hospitals.

SUMMARY

• Germs were known to cause disease – and doctors knew which germs caused which diseases. This led to drugs being developed to fight certain diseases. Vaccinations were also developed.

• Antiseptics and anaesthetics were developed to combat the problems of pain and infection during operations. This allowed more complicated surgery to take place.

• The government began to take some responsibility for the health of its citizens and introduced many public health reforms.

• Hospitals were improving and there were special schools for training nurses.

A Simple Guide To Mind Mapping

So what's a mind map?

Mind mapping is a special way of taking notes. Mind maps use only key words, phrases and images. They are quick to make, and because they look so interesting, many people find the information contained in them much easier to remember than other ways of making notes.

Why mind maps work

Mind maps helps you to quickly identify and understand the way pieces of the information fit together to build up the 'big picture'. They can help you revise all sorts of things, from detailed exam questions to whole topics.

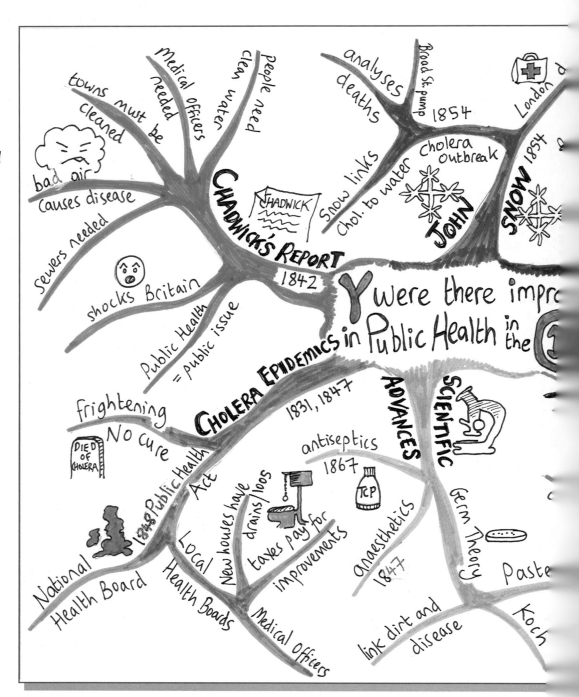

How to mind map

- Take a large sheet of paper and turn it to landscape.
- Write the topic/problem/question in the middle of the sheet and draw a frame around it. If you can make the centre a clear, strong visual image that fits in with the general theme of the mind map. When mind mapping 'Roman Medicine' for example make your central picture a Roman soldier's helmet perhaps!

- 'Branch Out' from the centre with the main ideas (like the branches of a tree) that you think about when looking at the central theme. Keep branching with each new 'association'.
- Put keywords on the lines – this helps reinforce your notes.
- Print, rather than write in your usual 'joined up' writing. This makes it easier to read and remember.
- Use **colour** to make things stand out. Things that stand out on the page will stand out in your mind.
- Use arrows, images and small (even silly) pictures wherever possible.
- Put down ideas as soon as they enter your mind – don't hold back. If you dry up in one area, move on to another branch – and if you run out of space, don't start a new sheet, just stick some paper on the side.
- Tony Buzan, one of the inventors of mind mapping, on www.mind-mapping.co.uk says: 'Have fun! Add a little humour, exaggeration or absurdity wherever you can. Your brain will delight in getting the maximum use and enjoyment from this process and will therefore learn faster, recall more effectively and think more clearly.'

Mind maps help you to break away from the 'normal' way or revising, which often consists of making long lists of facts. They are more compact than the typical way of making notes often taking up just one side of paper. And the way you complete them engages the creative part of your brain, helping you to write more freely and opening you up to new ways of thinking. Their colourful, interesting shape and structure stimulates your brain in to helping you to remember the information within it.

Why not try to mind map the following areas or questions:

- Egyptians • Greek medicine • Romans
- Hippocrates – how important was he?
- Renaissance medicine • Pasteur and Koch
- Germ Theory vs Four Humours
- Improvements in surgery

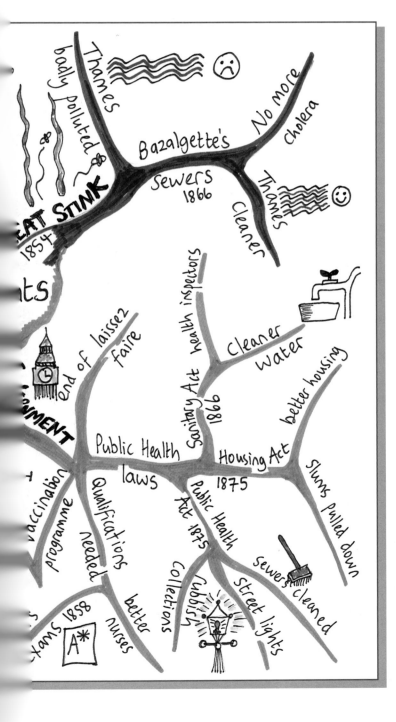

Why did fewer children die after 1900?

▸ Aim to understand why infant mortality decreased so much after 1900.

An adult's chance of a longer life improved sharply in the nineteenth century. Scientific progress and improved public health saw the average life expectancy go up from 30 years to about 50!

Those figures, of course, were for people who actually survived childhood. But surviving childhood was no easy matter. In fact, in 1900, the number of babies dying before they reached their first birthday was *higher* than it had been in 1800.

The worst year on record was 1899 when 163 babies out of every 1000 born died before they reached the age of one. And this was an *average* for the country as a whole – in some places it was much worse.

But these shocking **infant mortality** rates were as bad as they got. Steadily though, right up to the present day, the number of babies dying before their first birthday dropped – and more toddlers and children have survived childhood to reach adulthood.

So why did infant mortality decrease so much after 1900?

In 1899, a big army recruiting campaign took place to find men to fight in the Boer War in Africa. But army chiefs were alarmed by the fact that 40 out of every 100 young men who volunteered were unfit to be soldiers. And the army didn't have particularly high entry standards either! The government was so shocked too, that they set up a special committee to find out why so many men were so unsuitable. In 1904, the committee released their report – and amongst its many conclusions was the acknowledgement that many men were failing to get into the army because they had led such unhealthy childhoods (see **Source A**).

Source A ▾ *Many conclusions of the Committee on Physical Deterioration, 1904. Note the numerous references to children.*

- Bad health is not inherited; it can be improved by changes in food, hygiene and clothing.

- To further improve the health of the nation, the Committee believes we must:
  - get rid of overcrowded housing
  - make sure buildings are built correctly
  - control smoke pollution
  - ensure regular inspections of school children
  - set up day nurseries for the infants of working mothers, run by local councils
  - ban the sale of tobacco to children.

- Also, too many babies die due to poor feeding by the mother. This Committee believes we must teach young girls how to feed and look after babies properly.

The report came at a time when more and more people were beginning to feel that one of the key responsibilities of any government was to look after people who can't look after themselves. These people, including many politicians from the Liberal Party, believed that direct action from government was the way to improve the health and welfare of the nation. In 1906, the Liberal Party won the general election … and set to work.

In 1906, the School Meals Act allowed local councils to provide school meals, with poor children getting a free meal (see **Source B**). By 1914, over 158 000 children were having a free school meal every day. But lack of food was only part of the problem.

Source B ⮟ *Bradford was the first city to offer these meals. They were introduced at a time when politicians were reeling from research that showed that a poor child was, on average, 9cm shorter than a rich one.*

THIS WEEK'S MENU

Monday: Tomato soup – Currant roly-poly pudding

Tuesday: Meat pudding – Rice pudding

Wednesday: Yorkshire pudding, gravy, peas – Rice pudding and sultanas

Thursday: Vegetable soup – Currant pastry or fruit tart

Friday: Stewed fish, parsley sauce, peas, mashed potato – Blancmange

Source C ⮟ *This graph shows how children gained (and lost) weight during part of the year.*

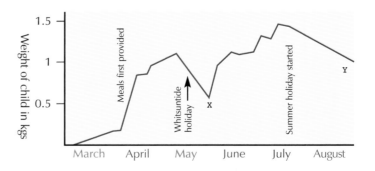

In 1907, the government told all councils that they should have a school medical service. At first, doctors examined the children and then parents paid for treatment. When lots of parents failed to follow through with treatment because they couldn't afford it, the government paid for school clinics to be set up where treatment was free (see **Source D**).

Source D ⮟ *An anxious mother watches the doctor examine her son in one of Britain's first free medical checks.*

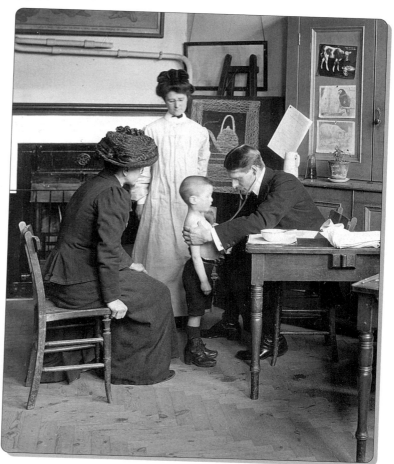

Other measures helped children. The Children and Young Person's Acts of 1908, for example, made children into 'protected persons', which meant that parents were breaking the law if they neglected their children (see **Source E**).

Source E ▾ *This was nicknamed 'The Children's Charter' and laid down in law many of the things that still protect children today.*

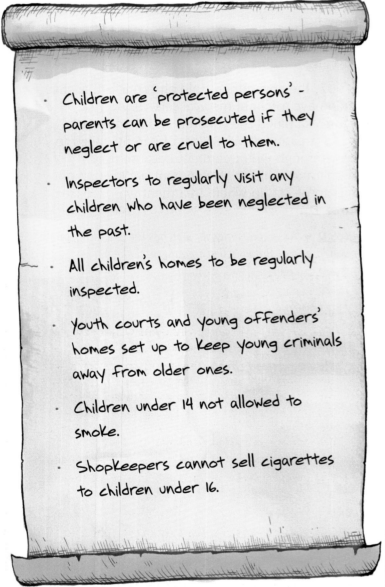

- Children are 'protected persons' - parents can be prosecuted if they neglect or are cruel to them.

- Inspectors to regularly visit any children who have been neglected in the past.

- All children's homes to be regularly inspected.

- Youth courts and young offenders' homes set up to keep young criminals away from older ones.

- Children under 14 not allowed to smoke.

- Shopkeepers cannot sell cigarettes to children under 16.

The school system was also seen as a way of improving children's health and well-being. From 1907, special schools were set up to teach young women about the benefits of breast feeding, hygiene and childcare.

Over the next 30 years, successive governments continued to take measures to improve the welfare of children (see **Source F**). Gradually, infant mortality began to drop … and drop … and drop (see **Source H**). A further boost to children's welfare was given in the 1940s with the introduction of the National Health Service (NHS). In fact, the care begins before the baby is born: a pregnant woman will get free treatment and advice at antenatal clinics, is given low-price milk and even maternity grants. Hospitals and nursing are free. When the baby is born, they receive cheap milk, food and vitamins, then a free education, cheap (or free) school meals, dental treatment and eye care. And if the child has any need that requires a special school because they are blind or deaf, for example, this costs the parent nothing! In 2002, the infant mortality rate was 5.2 per 1000 – that is, of every one thousand babies born, 5.2 die before they are a year old.

Source F ▾ *Dates in the health of children.*

1909: Overcrowded back-to-back housing banned. This is mainly a public health measure – but certainly improved the health of the children who would have had to live in the crowded, filthy, disease-ridden slums.

1918: Local councils to provide health visitors, clinics for pregnant women and day nurseries.

1919: Local councils to build new houses for poorer families.

1930: Huge slum clearance programme, again improving the lifestyle of the children who lived in them.

TOP EXAM TIP

Note how government action plays a key role in the decline of child deaths after 1900.

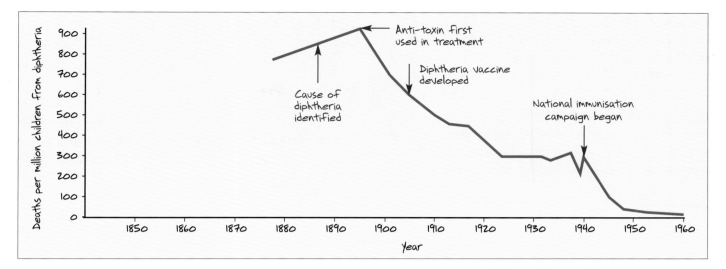

Source G ▲ *Diphtheria (a fever that makes a sufferer short of breath) killed many children in the nineteenth century. In 1940, the government introduced a campaign to get all children immunised.*

Source H ▼ *A graph to show infant mortality, 1840–2000.*

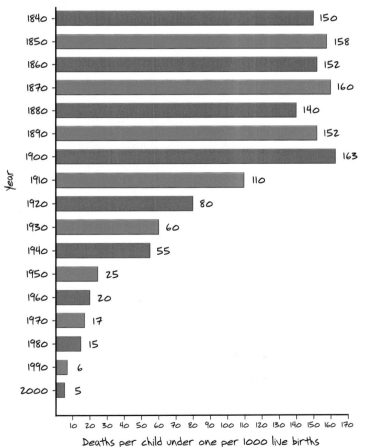

Deaths per child under one per 1000 live births

WISE UP WORD

- infant mortality

WORK

1 Look at **Source A**.
   a Why was the Committee on Physical Deterioration set up?
   b How did the report suggest that health could be improved?
   c Some historians think the report put an unfair blame on mothers. Do you agree?

2 Look at **Source B**.
   a Why were menus like this introduced in schools in the early 1900s?
   b Write down at least two reasons why many viewed this as a healthy menu.
   c Choose any day from the menu and write a few sentences comparing it to the menu you ate for dinner either today or another school day. You might wish to make a judgement about which was the healthier meal – yours or one a young person would have had in 1906.
   d In what ways have modern government today tried to improve the eating habits of young people at school?

3 Look at **Source C**.
   a What was the result of introducing school meals?
   b Why do you think children lost weight at points X and Y?

4 Apart from the introduction of school meals, how else were children helped in the early 1900s?

5 Look at **Source G**. Why do you think a national immunisation campaign for diphtheria was started in 1940?

6 Write an essay entitled 'Why did the infant mortality rate drop between 1900 and 1945?' It should be no more than 250 words long. Your teacher will help you to plan your answer.

Case study: The Penicillin story

> These pages will help you understand what "magic bullets" are, and how several different factors combined in the discovery and development of penicillin.

During the 1800s, scientists and doctors worked very hard to discover the causes of lots of different diseases. When the disease-carrying germs were discovered, they began looking at ways to *prevent* people from getting the diseases … and *cure* people who already had them. These two lines of research – prevention and cure (see boxes below) – led to some dramatic advances in the understanding of health and medicine.

PREVENTION: When Pasteur published his Germ Theory in 1861, the world began to realise that tiny creatures, called bacteria, were the cause of many diseases … and not bad air, cats and dogs or God's punishment. After Pasteur and Koch identified different bacteria which caused specific diseases. Pasteur found ways of using weakened forms of bacteria to allow the body to build up a resistance (or immunity) to the disease if it struck again (something successfully tried – but not understood by – Edward Jenner (smallpox) in 1796). Soon vaccines (as they became known) were perfected to prevent diseases such as diphtheria, TB, rabies and anthrax.

CURE: Koch found that certain coloured dyes 'sought out and found' specific bacteria in the body. His assistant, Paul Ehrlich, dreamed of finding a dye that would not only stain a specific bacterium – but kill it too! He widened his search, trying all sorts of chemicals in the hope that they would kill different bacteria – and if he found any, he said they would call them 'magic bullets'.

In 1909, Ehrlich and his team found a chemical that killed the bacteria that caused syphilis – a nasty STI that sometimes led to heart failure and blindness. The chemical was called Salverson and it was their 606th effort to produce a compound that killed syphilis and left human cells undamaged. It was soon known as Salverson 606.

Over the next 20 years, scientists found other '**magic bullets**', notably Prontosil, a red dye that worked against the germs that caused blood poisoning. Prontosil's active ingredient was sulphonamide (a chemical from coal tar) and soon more 'magic bullets' or 'sulpha drugs' had been developed to cure or control meningitis, pneumonia and scarlet fever.

By the 1920s, one nasty germ in particular remained undefeated by any magic bullet. No dye or chemical compound could be found to kill it. Its name was staphylococcus – a highly resistant form of bacteria that had over 30 different strains. It caused a wide range of illnesses and diseases, notably different types of food and blood poisoning, a variety of diseases and their horrid infections.

But a way to kill staphylococcus was close at hand. Scientists had known since the 1870s that some moulds (yes, the stuff that grows in an unwashed coffee cup or on your wet football boots after a week out in the rain!) could kill germs. So, in short, some kinds of bacteria (mould is a type of bacteria) killed other bacteria. One type of mould – penicillin to be precise – proved especially good at killing staphylococcus. Its discovery, and the eventual development of penicillin as the world's first and most famous **antibiotic** is a fascinating story. It's a tale of chance, individual brilliance, war, superb science and terrific technology. As you work through this case study, try to look out for each of the complex factors that contributed to the penicillin story.

Discovery

The penicillin mould was first discovered by a scientist in the 1870s called John Sanderson who noticed that very little grew near it. A few years later, Joseph Lister noticed the same thing … and took it one step further when he used it to treat a young nurse who had an infected wound. But Lister didn't get his notes published and took it no further. During World War One, a **bacteriologist** called Alexander Fleming was sent by St Mary's Hospital in London to study the treatment of wounded soldiers … and many were suffering from the ill effects of the staphylococcus germ! As ordinary chemical antiseptics were not working on some of the deeper wounds, Fleming saw at first hand the agony suffered by the soldiers (see **Source A**). When he retired from the war, he became determined to find a better way to treat their infected wounds.

Source A ▾ *From W Howard Hughes,* Alexander Fleming and Penicillin, *1974.*

"I remember being told to use antiseptics in the dressing of wounds – carbolic acid, boric acid and peroxide of hydrogen. But I could see for myself that these antiseptics did not kill all the microbes."

In 1928, Fleming was working on the hard-to-kill staphylococcus germs. When he went on holiday, he left several plates of the germs on a bench. When he came home, he noticed a large blob of mould in one of the dishes. Upon investigation, he noticed that the staphylococcus germs next to the mould had been killed. An excited Fleming took a sample of the mould … and found it to be our old friend, the penicillin mould. It appears that a spore from a penicillin mould grown in a room directly above Fleming's had floated down into his laboratory.

Fleming realised the germ-killing abilities of penicillin and published his findings. He concluded that penicillin was a natural antiseptic that killed many germs (he wrote a list) but did not harm living cells. He even grew lots of the penicillin mould, produced a juice from it and used it to clear up an infection in another scientist's eye (see **Source B**)!

Source B ▾ *Alexander Fleming.*

"Penicillin may be an efficient antiseptic for application to, or injection into, areas infected with penicillin-sensitive microbes. It is likely that penicillin will be used in the treatment of septic wounds."

But Fleming didn't inject penicillin into infected animals; he only used it as an antiseptic. As a result, few people regarded it as a major breakthrough and gradually even Fleming himself lost interest in it.

However, the penicillin story didn't end there. Soon, other key factors played a role in its success.

DEVELOPMENT

In the 1930s, a research team from Oxford University began compiling a list of all natural substances that could kill germs. They got hold of Fleming's article on penicillin and began to get very excited. Two of the scientists – Howard Florey and Ernst Chain – applied to the government for some money to begin further research into the germ-killing powers of penicillin. But they received only £25, not nearly enough to even start their research properly. In fact, they were probably lucky to get £25 – the British government, by 1939, was far more interested in World War Two that had just started. However, Florey and Chain pressed on and despite the fact that penicillin is extremely difficult to make, they managed to produce enough to successfully test on eight mice.

Their next move was to test it on humans – but they hadn't got enough because they needed 3000 times the amount of what they had used on the mice. So, over a couple of months, the two scientists turned their university department into a penicillin-producing factory. Using old milk bottles, hospital bedpans and a drug bath in which to grow the bacteria, they slowly collected enough penicillin to use on one human.

A 43-year-old policeman, Albert Alexander, was selected because all other drugs had failed on him. He had been scratched by a rose bush and a nasty infection had spread all over him. He had boils all over his body, on his lungs and one of his eyes had been removed. When he was injected with penicillin, the infection began to clear up. Tragically too, after five days, the penicillin ran out and the patient died ... but the success of penicillin had been noted by all involved. The next step was to try to work out how to produce masses of it!

MASS PRODUCTION

World War Two was a vital factor in transforming the supply of penicillin. The growing number of casualties meant that more penicillin was needed ... and quickly. In June 1941, Florey went to America to ask for help. The US government, realising the life-saving properties of this 'new' wonder treatment, agreed to pay several huge chemical companies to make millions of gallons of it in enormous vats. In 1943, there were stacks to treat only 1000 patients. By 1944, there was enough to treat 40 000 cases. By the end of the war, 250 000 soldiers were being treated – and the drug companies were able to use their production methods to begin making it for public use after the war was over.

IMPACT

During World War Two, officials estimated that about 15 per cent of wounded soldiers could have died without penicillin to fight their infections. Also, thousands and thousands of injured soldiers returned to battle much quicker than they would have done without their penicillin treatment. After the war, penicillin became available for doctors to use as a treatment for their patients – it was called an antibiotic and has saved the lives of millions of people. Indeed, unless you have an allergy to penicillin (around 10% of people do), almost all of you will probably have been prescribed penicillin by a doctor at some time. Penicillin has been said to treat bronchitis, gonorrhoea, impetigo, pneumonia, syphilis, tonsillitis, meningitis, septicaemia, septic arthritis, urine infection, boils, abscesses and all kinds of wounds.

Other antibiotics followed – streptomycin (1944), for example, proved an excellent treatment for tuberculosis whilst tetracycline (1953) was great for cleaning up skin infections and mitomycin (1956) is a chemotherapy drug that is given as a treatment for several different types of cancer.

TOP EXAM TIP

If you are asked about the importance of an individual (like Fleming) in the development of medicine, always compare their importance to other factors like war, science, chance and government action.

FACT *How much?*

70%, yes 70%, of all living things on planet earth are classed as 'bacteria'.

Who though?

If one of the questions on any major TV game show was 'Who developed penicillin?', the answer would almost definitely be 'Alexander Fleming'! This is due to the very well-known story of the mould floating into his laboratory and attacking the bacteria on his germ dish. But is this entirely true? Fleming certainly didn't discover penicillin, nor did he first use it to treat an infected wound (Lister did, remember – but didn't publish his notes).

Fleming <u>did</u> carry out detailed experiments and published his findings on penicillin's ability to kill germs – but he didn't try injecting penicillin into animals and he certainly didn't try it on humans.

Perhaps Howard Florey and Ernst Chain should be included in any answer to the question 'Who developed penicillin?' They were the first to develop a way to produce large quantities of the drug in huge vats using the latest technology ... and were the first to inject it directly into the human body when they tried (unsuccessfully in the end because they ran out!) to cure the policeman, Albert Alexander. Indeed, the answer to the question 'Who developed penicillin?' still divides debate today (see **Source F**).

Source C ▾ *Alexander Fleming.*

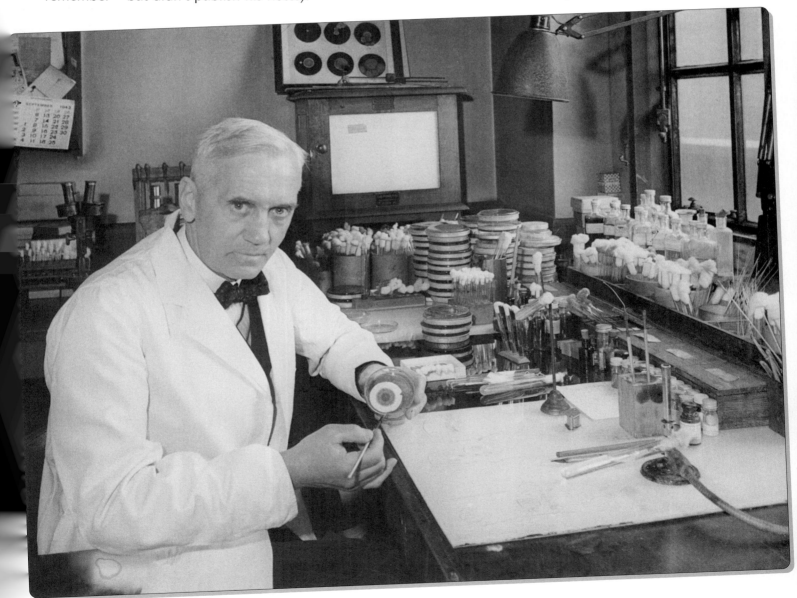

FACT *What next?*

There are now lots of new antibiotics coming on the market each year ... and they all work in basically the same way as penicillin – by killing bacteria. But they don't kill viruses (like HIV for example) so the search for other ways to kill and prevent viruses continues, vaccines against them being one of the main lines of research.

CLASSIC EXAM QUESTION

1 Briefly describe Fleming's work

2 Explain why penicillin was not developed before the 1940s

3 "The following were all equally important reasons why penicillin was developed:
   a The work of Fleming
   b The work of Florey and Chain
   c Chance
   d World War Two"

Do you agree with this statement?

Source D ⮯ *The Nobel Prize winners for 1945, including Alexander Fleming (second left) and Howard Florey (far right).*

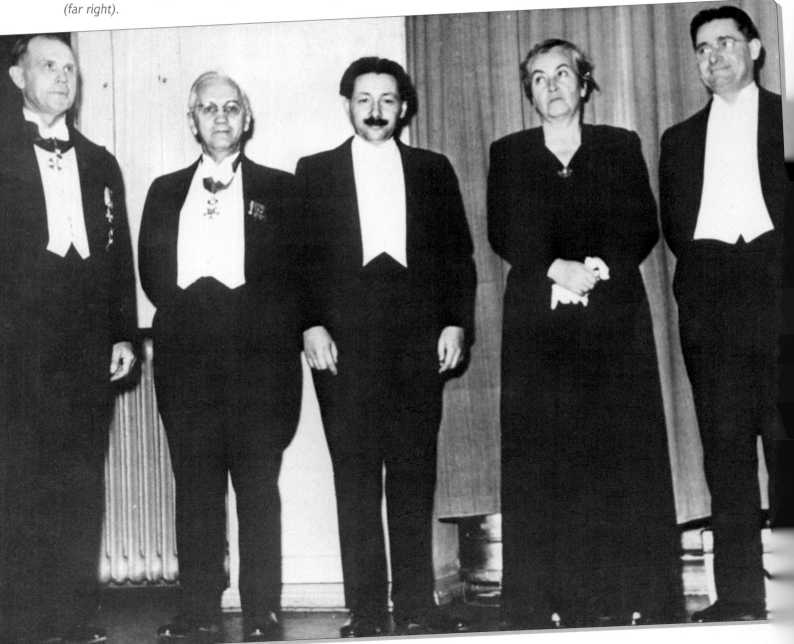

Source E ▾ *A description of the first use of penicillin by the British Army, 1943.*

"We had enormous numbers of infected wounded, terrible burn cases among the crews of the armoured cars. Sulphonamides had absolutely no effect on these cases. The last thing I tried was penicillin … the first man I tried it on was a young New Zealand officer called Newton. He had been in bed for six months with compound fractures of both legs. His sheets were soaked with pus and the heat of Cairo made it smell intolerable. Normally he would have died in a short time. I gave three injections a day of penicillin and studied the effects under the microscope … the thing seemed like a miracle. In ten days' time the leg was cured and in a month's time the young fellow was back on his feet. I had enough penicillin for ten cases. Nine out of ten of them were complete cures."

Source F ▾ *From Robert Hudson's* Disease and its Control *1983.*

"Fleming's role in the story of penicillin generally has been exaggerated … he was hampered by his inability to purify the substance, by his lack of chemical knowledge, and by his inability to find a collaborator with the requisite chemical knowledge … there is evidence that he was not convinced that the problem of isolating and purifying the active fraction of penicillin could be overcome … credit for purifying penicillin and for overcoming the many problems of mass production belongs to Howard Florey and his team of Oxford investigators, most notably Ernst Chain, who pointed the group towards penicillin in the first place."

Source G ▾ *Tony Triggs'* History of Medicine.

"After the war, Fleming worked in a hospital laboratory where he studied the sort of germs that had caused the battlefield deaths (and sometimes killed people who had operations). Fleming allowed his samples of germs to multiply in small glass dishes containing a jelly-like substance called agar. The germs spread over the surface of this agar. One day Fleming found that some mould was growing in one of the dishes and was killing the germs. He also found that preparations made from this mould killed most sorts of germs in the human body. This was the basis of a new drug known as *penicillin*. By the end of 1945, it had saved the lives of thousands of soldiers in World War Two."

WISE UP WORDS

antibiotic   bacteriologist   magic bullet

WORK

1 a Explain what is meant by the term 'magic bullet'.
  b How was Ehrlich's work different from Pasteur's?
2 Why is Fleming usually thought of as the discoverer of penicillin?
3 a Explain the part played in the penicillin story by:
   i) Joseph Lister   ii) Alexander Fleming
   iii) Florey and Chain   iv) Albert Alexander
   v) The US government.
  b How was the discovery of penicillin quickened by: i) luck   ii) war?
  c Who, or what, in your opinion, should get most credit for the discovery of penicillin? If you think one person or factor should get all the credit, explain why. However, if you think it is a combination of factors, explain why you think this and perhaps list the factors in order of importance.
4 a Explain what is meant by the term 'antibiotic'.
  b List some of the antibiotics mentioned in this chapter. State the approximate dates they were introduced and give an example of the sort of disease they fought.

'From the cradle to the grave'

Exam Focus

▸ Ensure you know:
* what health care was available before World War Two;
* why the National Health Service was introduced.

There is almost no one in Britain who isn't helped at some time or another by what is known as the **welfare state**. This is the name of the system by which the government aims to help those in need, mainly the old, the sick, unemployed and children. It is sometimes called 'social security' and aims to ensure that nobody goes without food, shelter, clothing, medical care, education or any other basic need because they can't afford it.

Study **Source A** carefully. It gives a basic outline of the welfare state. You and your family will almost certainly have been helped out by this system at one time or another.

Source A ▸ *The twentieth century saw the government accept the need to care for its citizens 'from the cradle to the grave'. This diagram explains how this was attempted.*

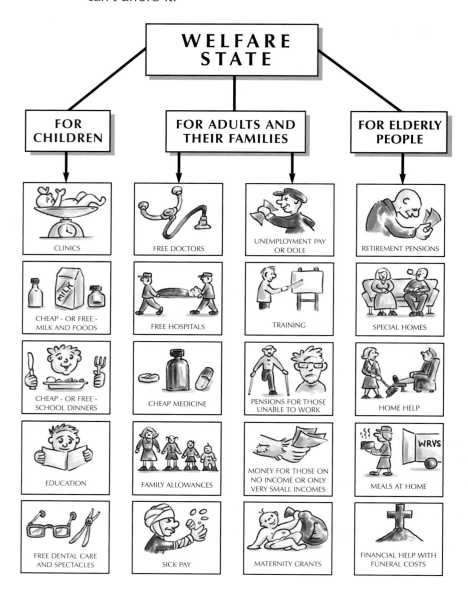

WELFARE STATE

FOR CHILDREN
- CLINICS
- CHEAP - OR FREE - MILK AND FOODS
- CHEAP - OR FREE - SCHOOL DINNERS
- EDUCATION
- FREE DENTAL CARE AND SPECTACLES

FOR ADULTS AND THEIR FAMILIES
- FREE DOCTORS
- FREE HOSPITALS
- CHEAP MEDICINE
- FAMILY ALLOWANCES
- SICK PAY

- UNEMPLOYMENT PAY OR DOLE
- TRAINING
- PENSIONS FOR THOSE UNABLE TO WORK
- MONEY FOR THOSE ON NO INCOME OR ONLY VERY SMALL INCOMES
- MATERNITY GRANTS

FOR ELDERLY PEOPLE
- RETIREMENT PENSIONS
- SPECIAL HOMES
- HOME HELP
- MEALS AT HOME (WRVS)
- FINANCIAL HELP WITH FUNERAL COSTS

Although we take things outlined in **Source A** for granted today, it is not a system that has been in place for many years. From 1906, the government had introduced *some* help for the most vulnerable sections of society – free school meals for poorer children, free school medical check-ups and treatment, small old-age pensions for the over 70s and basic sick and 'dole' pay – but nothing on the same scale as what was introduced after World War Two.

Source B ▼ *Speaking in 2006, Ivy Green from Nottingham remembers medical care in the 1930s.*

"You paid National Insurance as soon as you got a job. We called it 'the stamp' and it worked like any insurance policy does today. You paid a set amount each week into a central fund and this entitled you to some basic sick pay and care from a 'panel doctor' if you were ill … but because you only paid your 'stamp' if you had a job, it meant you missed out on doctor's care when you lost your job. So when there was high unemployment in the 1930s, loads of people were unable to get any medical treatment 'cos they hadn't been paying their stamp.

You could pay for a doctor to visit you – six pence I think. It wasn't a lot of money but still made you think twice about calling him. I'm sure lots of people mustn't have bothered to call a doctor 'cos of the money and let their illnesses go undiagnosed."

Towards the end of the war, a man named Sir William Beveridge wrote a report about the state of Britain. It outlined some of the problems that Britain would have to face once the war was over and suggested ways to improve things. In a Britain where people hoped that life would be better once the war was over, it became a surprise best seller.

As the war ended, an election was held to decide who would run the country after the war. The Labour Party promised to follow Beveridge's advice but the Conservative Party, led by Winston Churchill, refused to make such a promise. The Labour Party won the election easily – and Winston Churchill, the man who had led Britain during the war, was out of power!

Almost immediately, the new Labour government began to put Beveridge's plan into practice. Beveridge's reforms included:

- A National Health Service (NHS) was set up to provide health care for everyone. This made all medical treatment – doctors, hospitals, ambulances, dentists and opticians – free to all who wanted it. The scheme was opposed by doctors who didn't want to come under government control. The Minister of Health won them over by promising them a salary and allowing them to treat private patients as well.
- A weekly family allowance payment was introduced to help with child care costs.
- The very poor received financial help or 'benefits'.
- The school leaving age was raised to 15 to give a greater chance of a decent education and more free university places were created.

Source C ▼ *From a 2004 interview with Frederick Rebman about the way hospital care was funded in the 1920s and 1930s.*

"I remember our panel doctor coming to visit me once because I had a suspected appendicitis. In the end, it was a false alarm but they still kept me in hospital for three days. When I came out they asked me for my father's details. We were in business you see and could afford a shilling or two so they asked my father for a contribution."

Source D ▶ *How medical care was funded in the 1930s.*

- The government's programme of 'slum clearance' continued as large areas of poor-quality housing were pulled down and new homes built. Twelve new towns were created and by 1948, 280 000 council homes were being built each year.

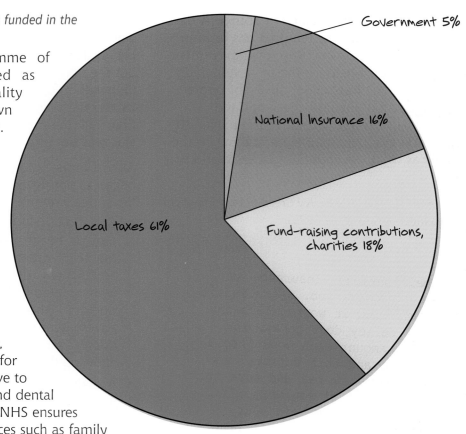

Government 5%

National Insurance 16%

Local taxes 61%

Fund-raising contributions, charities 18%

Of course, all this cost money. All workers had to pay for the service through taxation and over the years, the cost of welfare state services like the NHS had rocketed (see **Source G**). In fact, the NHS itself did not stay free for long. Working people today have to pay for doctors' prescriptions and dental treatment for example, but the NHS ensures that no one is deprived of services such as family planning, physiotherapy, child care, cancer screening, asthma clinics and minor surgery because they can't afford it.

However, the NHS is rarely out of the news, mainly due to the fact that it has problems: waiting lists seem to be getting longer and doctors and nurses are overworked. There is rarely a month that goes by without some big media scandal about 'dirty wards', 'crumbling hospitals' or 'nurses doing long hours'. The main problem, of course, is money. Modern drugs are very expensive and modern medicine means that people are living longer … so there are more elderly people than ever before – and older people use the NHS more than younger people. The NHS has always been, and should continue to be, a really hot topic in British society!

> **TOP EXAM TIP**
>
> *Make sure you can explain why the NHS was introduced.*

Source E ▼ *From a speech made by Aneurin Bevan, the man appointed by the government to introduce the NHS. It seems that Bevan's words hit home with health care providers – women's needs became a priority and they are now four times more likely to consult a doctor than men. Life expectancy for women has risen from 66 to 78 since 1948.*

"A person ought not to be stopped from seeking medical assistance by the anxiety of doctors' bills … medical treatment should be made available to treat rich and poor alike in accordance with medical need and no other criteria. Worry about money in a time of sickness is a serious hindrance to recovery apart from its unnecessary cruelty. Records show that it is the mother in the average family who suffers most from the absence of a full health service. In trying to balance her budget she puts her own needs last."

Source F ▼ *From an interview with Frederick Rebman, speaking in 2004, remembering the introduction of the NHS.*

"We were sorry to see Churchill voted out, he was our war leader, but he never promised to give the new ideas a go. The Labour Party did you see, and they publicised this in all the papers … servicemen [men in the army, navy and air force] like me expected so much after the war, perhaps Utopia [a perfect world], and the welfare state seemed to be a good start. I didn't mind the idea of paying a bit more of my salary to know that a doctor or a dentist was there if I needed them. I felt it was worth it, that the government cared about us a bit more I suppose … I think there was a bit of a rush when the NHS first started. There were stories of people going and getting whole new sets of teeth, new glasses, even wigs. Perhaps they'd have struggled on before with their short-sightedness or their painful teeth, but now they didn't have to."

Source H ▼ *A letter to the Daily Mail, November 2006. The expense and organisation of the NHS still attracts fierce debate today.*

"International Health Service

I'm a doctor who was working at a major London hospital last Monday.

I treated patients from Portugal, Ecuador, Mexico, Albania, Peru, Algeria, Italy, Germany, Ethiopia, Eritrea, Iran and Iraq. There was also one from England.

The problem with the NHS isn't about too little money, but too many international patients who come here and get free treatment without any questions being asked of them."

WISE UP WORD

- welfare state

Source G ▼ *The cost of the NHS, 1948–1992.*

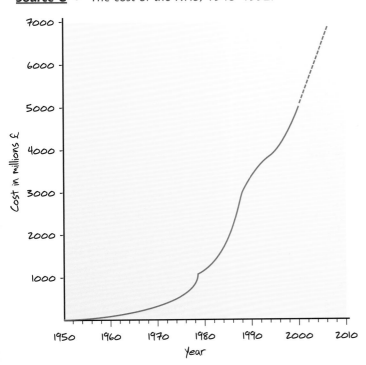

Cost in millions £ / Year

WORK

1 In your own words, describe how the most vulnerable people in society were looked after before World War Two.

2 **a** Explain what is meant by the term 'welfare state'.
   b What was the Beveridge Report?
   c Why were some doctors against the NHS when it was proposed in the Beveridge Report?
   d How did Beveridge win them over?

3 Look at **Source E**.
   a Who was Aneurin Bevan?
   b What point does he make about women in his speech?

4 Look at **Source F**.
   a According to the source, why did the Labour Party win the election in 1945?
   b Why do you think people rushed out to get 'whole new sets of teeth, new glasses, even wigs' when the NHS first started?

5 Why do you think the NHS is such a controversial topic still today?

What's up Doc?

Topic Focus

> Aim to remember at least 5 ways in which a doctor's role has changed in the last 150 years.

Exam Focus

> To know how the training and role of doctors has changed in the last 150 years.

The 'Family Doctor' or **General Practitioner** (GP) is one of the best-known and most respected roles in communities all over Britain. They are often seen as a 'fount of all knowledge' when it comes to diagnosing and treating illness and, for most people, the local GP is the first place they go when they feel really poorly. So how has the role of the local doctor developed? What are their key duties and responsibilities in today's society? And how has the training and role of doctors changed in recent centuries? Read the 'case files' of the following doctors carefully. They outline the key changes in their roles and training over the last 150 years. You will be asked to complete a comparison table on page 137.

The birth of the family doctor

It was not until the early 1800s that doctors first began to take exams for their certificates in medicine and some hospitals opened specialist schools to train them. In 1858 a new law (the General Medical Act) stated that there should be a General Medical Council (GMC) and all qualified doctors had to put their names on the general medical register. There were 15 000 names on the register by 1860. By then any new doctors had to have passed exams on anatomy, physiology, pharmacy, surgery and midwifery – and when qualified they became known as 'general practitioners', or as they usually preferred to call themselves, 'doctors'.

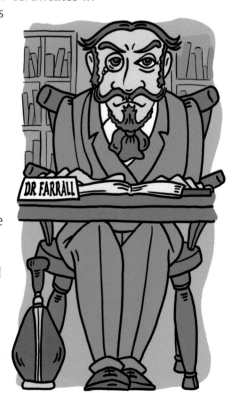

Dr Farrall (1860)

- Lots of hands on training in hospitals.
- Basic scientific knowledge, exam certificates to prove it.
- Very little useful equipment.
- Highly respected in the community.
- Little understanding of the real cause of the disease, Pasteur's 'Germ theory' hasn't been published yet!
- Not paid by the government, relies on payments from his patients.
- Recently started a 'sick club' in the local town to attract poorer patients – he charges a few shillings for a year's treatment.
- Will visit wealthy patients in their own homes.
- Doesn't know any woman doctors – they are not allowed at this time.

Dr Edwards (1930)

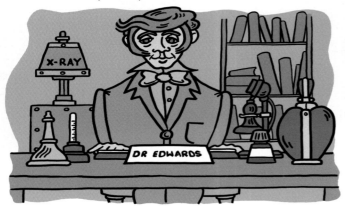

- Has some understanding of the causes of illness and disease.
- Highly respected in the community.
- Can offer few cures, but diphtheria and TB vaccines have been developed by now. This means that the number of deaths from these two major killer diseases has started to decline.
- Not paid by the government, relies on payments from his patients. Sees some patients for free.
- Will visit wealthy patients in their own homes.
- Some of his income comes from being 'on the panel'. This means that he is part of a group (or panel) of doctors who will treat patients who have paid into a sort of insurance scheme, similar to a 'sick club'.
- He knows a few female doctors, but not many.
- Can refer patients to expensive specialists if they have enough money to pay them.
- Basic equipment – a thermometer, stethoscope, perhaps an X-ray machine.

Dr Wilson (2009)

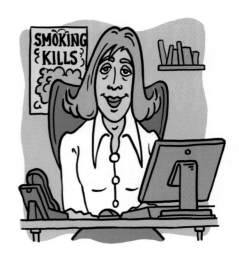

- Paid a salary by the government, patients do not pay directly anymore.
- Sees most of her patients in the surgery, but is 'on call' some of the time too. This means she has to work through the night or over a weekend occasionally.
- Understands many of the causes of disease and can offer all sorts of cures.
- Can use the latest technology to diagnose illnesses.
- Can refer patients to specialists in large hospitals for diagnosis and/or treatment.
- Is as likely to be a woman as a man.
- Educated at university for many years, as well as practical experience in hospitals.
- Still highly respected, but perhaps not as much as in previous times – patients expect a far higher standard of care than ever before.
- Works hard with patients on 'prevention' of illness rather than just 'cures'. This includes talking to patients about the benefits of a healthy lifestyle as well as other important issues like immunising children and older people against illness.

WORK

1 Copy and complete a table similar to the one here.

	Dr Farrall	Dr Edwards	Dr Wilson
Training			
How they are paid			
Respect in community			
Understanding of causes of illness			
Cures available			
Number of female doctors			
Equipment			
Ability to treat poorer patients			
Use of specialists			

2 Choose three areas where you think a doctor's life has changed a lot. Try to suggest reasons for these changes.

Into the twentieth century

Exam Focus

▸ For exam practice try to learn:
- five ways in which medical knowledge has improved since 1900;
- five ways in which surgery has improved since 1900;
- five ways in which treatment has improved since 1900.

Massive changes had taken place in the years up to 1900. More than ever before was known about the causes of diseases and the way to prevent some of them. The government too had started to take more responsibility for the health of its citizens by clearing the worst of the overcrowded slum areas of the dirtiest towns, building proper sewer systems and laying new water pipes.

But despite all the important changes of the 1800s, life expectancy for the average man still lay at the lowly age of 46 (50 for a woman), over 160 out of every 1000 babies born died before their first birthday and doctors were often still unable to cure their patients as there was no effective way to fight internal infection. Operations too, were still incredibly dangerous. Despite the widespread use of anaesthetics and antiseptics, post-operation infection still remained a major drawback.

But the twentieth century saw an explosion in scientific and medical discoveries and developments which proved significant in achieving a fuller understanding of health and medicine than ever before.

Now study the timeline carefully. It charts some of the most significant changes in the fields of medical knowledge about the body and disease, surgery and treatment.

■ **1895: X-rays** discovered by a German called Wilhelm Röntgen. He used his wife's hand for the first pictures. For the first time, doctors could get information about the insides of patients' bodies without cutting them open.

● **1896:** Hospitals installed the first X-ray machines and in America, a doctor named Walter Cannon used a **barium meal** with an X-ray to track the passage of food through a patient's troubled digestive system.

● **1898:** Polish scientists Marie and Pierre Curie discovered the element radium. It was soon found that radium destroyed diseased cells and so was used in cancer therapy. It was called **radiotherapy**. What wasn't known at the time was that, without protection, radium could make the air radioactive, cause radiation sickness and permanently damage the body. Marie Curie died of leukaemia after working for 25 years handling radioactive material.

● **1900:** More and more was discovered about vitamins – which allowed doctors to prescribe them to cure illnesses like beriberi, rickets, pellagra and anaemia.

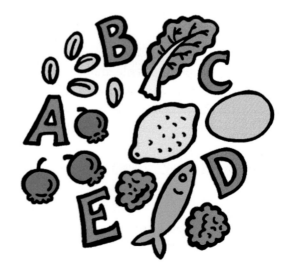

■ **1901:** Scientist Landsteiner discovered there are different blood groups. This meant that the blood of the recipient could be matched carefully to that of the donor to reduce the chance of new blood being rejected.

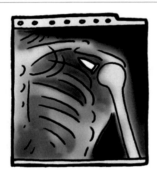

● **1910:** British scientist Henry Dale discovered the chemical histamine, which is produced by the body during an allergic reaction. This allowed scientists to understand allergic reactions and work on a cure. Ever taken 'anti-histamine' tablets for hay fever?

▲ **1914:** Mobile X-ray units were used during World War One to, among other things, find bullets in wounded soldiers.

● **1914:** Albert Hustin added glucose and sodium citrate to blood so it can be stored for longer periods of time (it just clotted and hardened before). Now wounded soldiers, for example, fighting in World War One, could get the blood they needed quickly.

■ **1921:** Frederick Banting and Charles Best discovered insulin, which breaks down sugar in the blood stream. As a result, they found the cause of diabetes and were able to treat it.

■ **1923:** American Edgar Allen discovered oestrogen (the hormone that powers 'femaleness').

● **1928:** Penicillin's properties as a disease killer were identified by Scottish bacteriologist Alexander Fleming by chance. Penicillin became the first antibiotic.

■ **1931:** The invention of the electron microscope allowed doctors to see some types of bacteria and viruses for the first time.

■ **1935:** Ernst Laqueur identified testosterone, the hormone that powers 'maleness'.

▲ **1940:** British surgeon Archie McIndoe surgically rebuilt the faces of airmen burned in their planes during World War Two. This was the first plastic surgery – and by 2000, over six million cosmetic surgery operations were performed in the USA alone.

▲ **1944:** The first eye bank was opened in New York. Eyes can only be stored for a short time before they become useless.

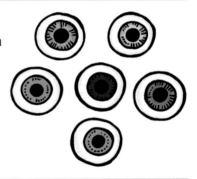

▲ **1950:** Canadian surgeon William Bigelow performed the first open-heart surgery to repair a 'hole' in a baby's heart.

■ **1951:** Mexican company Syntex developed norethisterone – a man-made hormone that prevents women ovulating. This led to the production of the first contraceptive pill.

▲ **1952:** First miniature hearing aid produced.

▲ **1952:** First kidney transplant.

■ **1953:** Scientists Francis Crick and James Watson discovered DNA (see Fact box). The understanding of DNA could lead to such developments as gene therapy, genetic screening and genetic engineering.

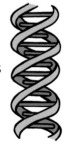

FACT *'It's in your genes'*

DNA – or deoxyribonucleic acid – is in every cell in our body. Think of DNA as a long list of instructions or a code that operates every one of these cells ... and there are 3000 million letters in the code. The instructions are grouped together in **genes** and each gene has a different function. Some genes decide on your eye colour or how tall you will be. Others decide whether you will develop a disease or a disability ... and some genes can be passed from parent to child.

Since the early twentieth century, scientists knew that DNA existed – an expert in X-rays called Rosalind Franklin even photographed it in 1951 – but she couldn't identify the structure. In 1953, two scientists at Cambridge University – Crick and Watson – successfully mapped out DNA and proved it was present in every cell in the body and could pass information from one generation to the next.

■ **1953:** American Leroy Stevens discovered stem cells. These are the essential cells common in multi-cellular organisms. They are able to renew themselves and can also differentiate into specific cell types.

▲ **1961:** First pacemaker fitted – a mechanical device that maintains a regular heartbeat.

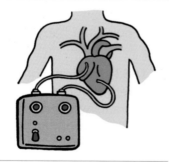

▲ **1962:** Surgeons at a hospital in America re-attached the arm of a 12-year-old boy.

▲ **1963:** First liver transplant.

▲ **1967:** Christian Barnard, a South African heart surgeon, performed the first heart transplant. The patient lived for 18 days. In 2002, there were over 2000 heart transplants performed in the USA – 87% of the patients lived for at least one year.

● **1970:** British scientist Roy Calne developed the drug cyclosporine which prevents the body rejecting transplanted organs.

▲ **1972:** British surgeon Sir John Charnley developed hip replacements.

■ **1973:** British scientist Geoff Hounsfield invented the CAT scanner, which uses X-ray images from many angles to build up a 3D image of the inside of the body.

■ **1975:** Endoscopes were developed. These are fibre optic cables with a light source that allow doctors to go into small cuts in the skin to 'see' inside the body.

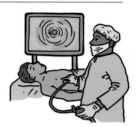

● **1978:** Throughout the 1970s, doctors had used IVF fertility treatment to help childless women become pregnant. In 1978, Louise Brown became the first 'test tube baby'. In 2005, a 66-year-old Romanian woman gave birth to twins through IVF.

▲ **1984:** At Harvard University in the USA, two burn victims were given skin grafts. The skin had been grown in a laboratory 'skin farm' from tiny pieces. One square centimetre had grown to half a square metre.

FACT *World Health Organization (WHO)*

A worldwide organization dedicated to improving health was set up after World War II in 1946. The aim of the World Health Organization is to help all the people of the world to reach the highest possible level of health. 'Health' was actually defined by them as 'the state of physical, mental and social well-being' and not just the absence of disease! In 1967, the WHO began a successful campaign to wipe out smallpox – and in 1980 after a huge vaccination programme, they announced that the disease had been eradicated across the world. Other programmes are underway to wipe out measles, whooping cough and polio. A global WHO programme is also currently underway to fight the spread of HIV and AIDS. According to the WHO's annual report in 2000, AIDS has become the fourth biggest killer in the world.

1986: British woman Davina Thompson became the first heart, lung and liver transplant patient.

1987: MRI scanning now widely used to monitor electrical activity of the brain.

1990: The **Human Genome Project** in the US mapped all the genes in the Human body – 100 000 of them – and identified their role. The money for this massive project came from the governments of the USA, Britain, Japan, France and Canada as well as drug companies that hoped to profit from developing drugs based on understanding DNA.

1997: Researchers in Scotland breed the first cloned animal – a sheep called Dolly. Dolly was cloned in 1996 from a cell taken from a six-year-old ewe. Cloning is the process of creating an identical copy of an original organism or thing. Dolly died in February 2003 from a lung disease.

2002: American surgeons implanted electrodes connected to a miniature computer into the visual cortex of a blind man. Using a video camera mounted onto his glasses, the man was able to 'see' well enough to drive a car.

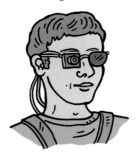

2006: First face transplant (see **Sources C** and **D** on page 130).

Timeline Key	
■	knowledge about body and disease
▲	surgery
●	treatment

Source A ▾ *A patient receives radiography treatment, 1920. The treatment can remove some cancerous growths from patients.*

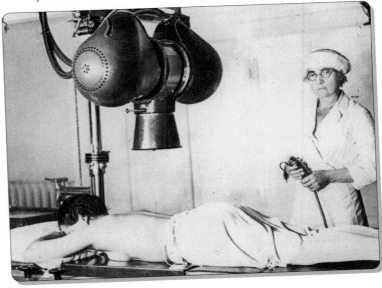

Source B ▾ *The use of an X-ray machine during World War One. Here it is being used to locate a bullet in a soldier's heart in 1915.*

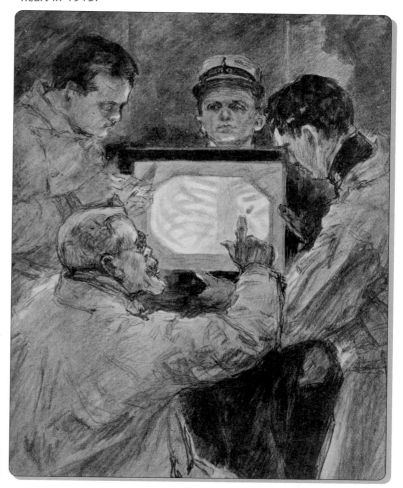

Source C ▶ A photograph of Isabelle Dinoire who received the world's first partial face transplant. In a 15-hour operation, surgeons used tissue, muscles, arteries and veins from a brain-dead woman to rebuild Dinoire's face. Dinoire, who was attacked by a dog, is from Lille, France.

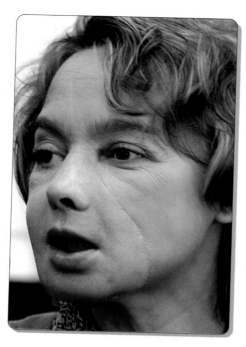

Source D ▶ Here, the surgeons explain how they are to perform the face transplant in a press conference in 2005.

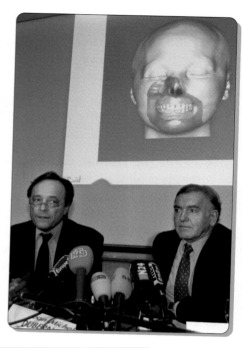

Individual brilliance
As across all periods of history, the twentieth century saw some geniuses in action: Curie, Fleming, Crick and Watson for example.

Attitudes and government
Modern politicians have realised that one of their main priorities is to help and protect the people they serve. Free health care and medical treatment, as well as massive government health education schemes (such as the 'Healthy Schools' project) are part of this.

Science and technology
New technology – such as keyhole surgery and X-ray machines for example – helped doctors and surgeons to develop new techniques for identifying illnesses and operating on them.
New discoveries, like DNA, have led to many new possibilities.

So why did health and medicine improve so much in the twentieth century?

War
Two world wars have meant that the government has spent a fortune on research testing so that the latest drugs and surgical techniques are available for wounded soldiers. Doctors have had to find better ways to treat casualties too, thus advancing medical knowledge. The development of blood transfusions during World War One is a good example of this.

Money
Governments spend far more money on research and care than ever before. For example, the government has a huge breast and cervical cancer screening programme which aims to identify illness before it develops. Drug companies too spend huge amounts on research and development hoping to make money from cures.

Communication
New ideas spread rapidly due to the increased use of television, the growth of newspapers and even the Internet. Huge TV and radio advertisements have made more people than ever before aware of health risks associated with smoking and alcohol for example.

Source E ▸ *IVF treatment – the moment of fertilisation. A doctor uses a hollow needle to inject a single sperm into an egg. This technique has only been made possible because of technological and scientific advances and inventions such as the hollow needle and electron microscopes.*

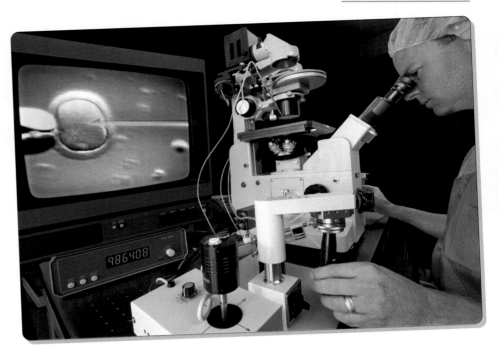

Source F ▾ *Francis Crick (right) and James Watson photographed in 1959. Their discovery of the structure of DNA was seen as a major medical breakthrough. The reason for this is down to the fact that many of today's most feared diseases – cancer and heart disease for example – are not like the most feared diseases of long ago. Most infectious diseases – smallpox, cholera, TB and so on – can be prevented or cured today. But doctors are still struggling with cancers and heart disease. Inherited diseases too, like Downs Syndrome or diabetes, have also stumped doctors and scientists – and cause much fear because they are <u>not</u> caused by germs that can be dealt with. Understanding DNA – and how our body works – may lead to a fuller understanding of diseases like cancer, heart disease, Downs Syndrome and many more … and if doctors understand them better, they are more equipped to prevent them or find cures.*

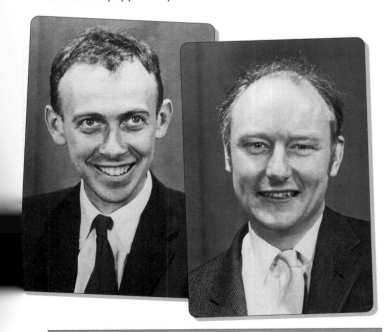

WISE UP WORDS

- barium meal   radiotherapy   DNA
  Human Genome Project   X-rays   IVF treatment

WORK

1. Look through the timeline on pages 138–141. Find five examples of ways in which developments in medical knowledge, surgery and treatment have affected <u>you</u> since you were born. For example, some of you will have benefitted from the effects of Henry Dale's discovery in 1910 of the chemical histamine during the summer hay fever season!

   Make a list of the ways in which twentieth century developments have benefitted <u>your</u> health.

2. Find examples on the timeline that show how medical progress has been affected by:
   - war   • governments   • science and technology
   - individual brilliance   • chance.

3. Write a sentence or two about the following:
   - radiotherapy   • IVF treatment   • DNA
   - Human Genome Project

4. Imagine you have to choose three medical developments from the twentieth century to include on a web page about 'The greatest advances in medical history'. Which three developments would you choose? Give reasons for your choices.

TOP EXAM TIP

Make sure you understand the importance of science and technology in the development of modern medicine. Remember though, that they have not been the only factors in changing medicine in the modern world.

How did two world wars change medicine?

Topic Focus

▶ Remember at least two examples of medical progress which resulted from World War One and two which resulted from World War Two.

Throughout history, one of the key times when the latest medical techniques and the most up-to-date medical technology is needed is during wartime. If the medical services are good, then more soldiers have a chance of survival, and the more soldiers there are available, the greater the country's chances of victory.

Medicine usually develops at a greater rate during wartime than in peace time. Governments of fighting countries pour a lot of money into developing ways of getting their injured soldiers back 'fighting fit' as soon as possible. Doctors and surgeons work even harder in wartime, often in battlefield situations to develop their ideas in order to treat the injured. The huge numbers of wounded soldiers give doctors and surgeons more opportunity than is available in peace time.

The two world wars that took place during the 20th century were huge conflicts which killed and wounded millions more people than in any wars before them. New and deadly weapons – high explosive shells, gas bombs, hand grenades and machine guns – were used on a massive scale for the first time and inflicted terrible injuries. Over 10 million people were killed in World War One (1914–1918) and over 20 million in World War Two (1939–1945), and these figures do not include the huge amount of people who were injured ... and wars always tend to wound more than they can kill! Yet despite the great suffering caused by these two horrific wars, a number of improvements in medicine were made as a direct result.

Study the following cartoon labels carefully. They outline the impact on health and medicine brought about by World War One. Advances made during and as a result of World War Two are shown on the pages that follow.

What Medical Progress Did World War One Bring About?

Blood Transfusions

Although blood transfusions had been tried for centuries, it wasn't until 1900, when Karl Landsteiner discovered blood groups that scientists worked out how to do them successfully. They realised that a transfusion only worked if the donor's blood type matched the receiver's. Even then it wasn't possible to store blood for long because it clotted so quickly! As a result, many people still died from loss of blood – so a solution to the problem of storing blood was needed. In 1914, Albert Hustin discovered that glucose and sodium citrate stopped blood from clotting on contact with air. Other advances meant that blood could be bottled, packed in ice and taken to where it was needed by surgeons operating on soldiers.

Plastic Surgery

During World War One, the hard work and dedication of Harold Gillies, an army doctor, led to the development of what we now call 'plastic surgery'. He set up a special unit to graft skin and treat men suffering from severe facial wounds. He is commonly recognised as one of the first surgeons to consider a patient's appearance when treating their wounds. Queens Hospital in Kent opened in 1917 and provided over 1000 beds for soldiers with severe facial wounds by 1921. Over 5000 servicemen had been treated by 1921.

Broken Bones

New techniques were developed during World War One to repair broken bones. For example, the Army Leg Splint (or Keller-Blake Splint) was developed which elevated and extended the broken leg 'in traction'. This helped the bones knit together more securely. The splint is still in use today.

Shell Shock

The mental strain of war could cause shell shock. Some shell-shocked soldiers had panic attacks, others shook all the time or were unable to speak or move. To begin the army refused to believe that shell shock existed and many of the men were treated as cowards. However, by the end of the war there were so many cases that shell shock was officially recognised. Today the condition is known as PTSD, or Post-Traumatic Stress Disorder.

Infection

Battlefields are incredibly dirty places and lethal wound infections such as gangrene were common. Through trial and error, surgeons worked out that the best way to prevent this was to cut away any infected flesh and soak the wound in salty (saline) solution. This wasn't ideal, but as a short-term answer in a battle situation, it saved many lives.

X-rays

X-rays were discovered in 1895 and soon hospitals were using then to look for broken bones and disease. However, it was during World War One that they became really important. Mobile X-ray machines were used near the battlefield to find out exactly where in the wounded soldier's body bullets or piece of shrapnel had lodged without having to cut him wide open!

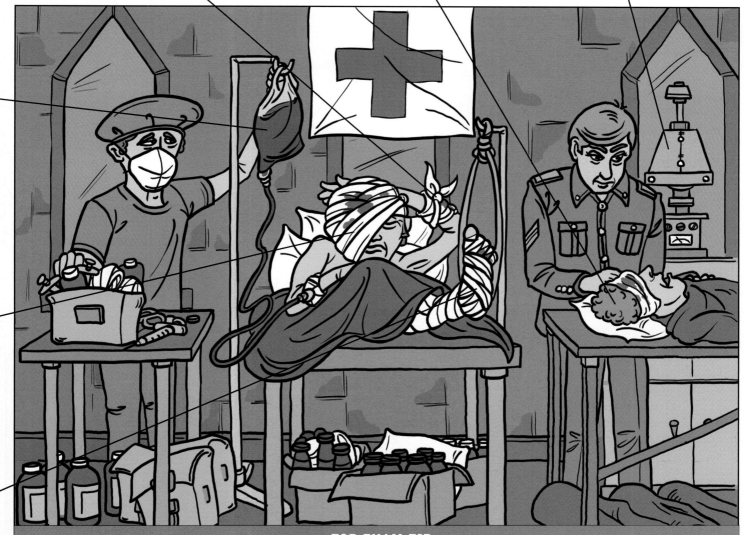

TOP EXAM TIP

A good GCSE student gives a balanced view. So whilst writing about the advances caused by war, remember that some historians have argued that World War One actually hindered the development of medicine in some ways. After all, thousands of doctors were taken away from their normal work to treat casualties, and lots of medical research was stopped.

So what was the impact of World War Two on medicine?

World War One speeded up developments in medicine that probably would have happened anyway. For example, scientists had been working on blood transfusions for many years, but the amount of blood needed by soldiers in World War One meant that scientists worked even harder and faster to make blood transfusions a success! X-rays too, had been discovered in 1895, but it was during World War One that they became really important.

It was a similar situation in World War Two. The millions of wounded soldiers meant that doctors, surgeons and scientists worked hard to develop new medicines and techniques – but they also tried to develop some of the advances made in earlier years. **Source A** sums up the impact of World War Two on medicine and health in Britain.

Source A ▼ *The impact of World War Two.*

Plastic surgery
A doctor from New Zealand, Archibald McIndoe (cousin of Harold Gillies), used new drugs (such as penicillin) to prevent infection when treating pilots with horrific facial burns. His work on reconstructing damaged faces and hands was respected all over the world.

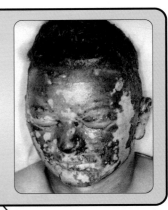

Blood transfusions
Advances in storing blood in the years after World War One meant it could be kept fresh and useable for longer. This led to the British National Blood Transfusion Service opening in 1938. Large blood banks were developed in both the USA and Britain during World War II, much of it donated by civilians.

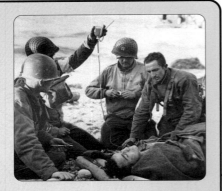

THE IMPACT OF WORLD WAR TWO

Heart surgery
Heart surgery progressed during World War Two. American army surgeon Dwight Harken cut into beating hearts and used his bare hands to remove bullets and bits of shrapnel. His findings helped heart surgery develop greatly after the war.

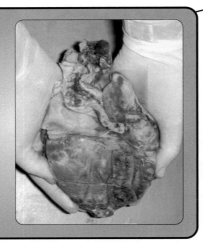

Diet
Shortages of some foods during the war meant that the government encouraged people to grow their own food. This actually improved people's diet because the food they encouraged civilians to grow – fresh vegetables for example – was very healthy!

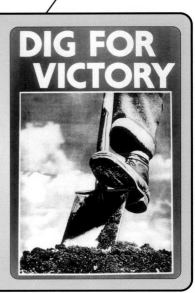

DIG FOR VICTORY

Hygiene and disease

In order to keep the nation 'fighting fit' posters were produced which encouraged people to keep healthy. They warned against the dangers of poor hygiene. A national immunisation programme against diphtheria (a bacterial infection which killed many children) was launched too.

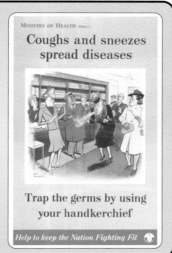

MINISTRY OF HEALTH says:—

Coughs and sneezes spread diseases

Trap the germs by using your handkerchief

Help to keep the Nation Fighting Fit

The National Health Service

When war broke out, the government increased its involvement in medical care. They knew there had to be adequate medical services to cope with the large number of casualties. Soon people started to think about how best to organise health care after the war on a national basis. In 1942 a civil servant named William Beveridge (pictured) proposed a 'free National Health Service for all' — and just after the war finished, the NHS was born.

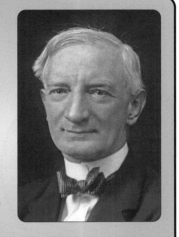

Poverty

During the war, over one million children were evacuated from the towns and the cities into the countryside. Many of the children were very poor and the cleaner, more nutritional, lifestyle they enjoyed in the countryside improved their health. The whole experience highlighted the levels of poverty endured by some children in Britain's towns and cities, and increased the government's commitment to improve things after the war.

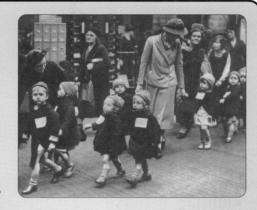

Drug development

Penicillin, the first antibiotic, was developed in the years leading up to the war. The British and American governments realised how important this new 'wonder drug' could be in curing infections in deep wounds. By 1944 enough penicillin was produced to treat all the Allied forces in Europe.

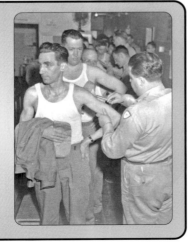

WORK

1 Explain why wars often result in major advances and developments in health and medicine?

2 Imagine you were an army surgeon in World War One. Write a short letter home to your friends and family explaining how the latest scientific and technological developments have helped you in your work.

3 a Look at **Source A**. Explain how each of the advances, ideas and developments improved medicine and health.

 b Which of these developments would not have happened if it wasn't for World War Two?

CLASSIC EXAM QUESTION

What impact did the two world wars have on medicine in the modern world?

Twenty-first century medicine

▶ Over the next 10 pages, you will learn about:
- some controversial developments in medicine;
- some of the latest techniques and advances in surgery;
- alternative medicines;
- medicine around the world.

In 2004, a group of scientists and doctors predicted that by 2104, the average age of death would be 100 (it stood at 81 for women and 76 for men in 2002). That's right – 100 years of age. They put this down to the advances made in medicine in the twentieth century – and the advances they believe will take place in the twenty-first.

So what can we expect? How will surgery develop? How will tomorrow's doctors fight today's diseases? And where do things like 'positive health' and 'alternative medicines' fit into the hi-tech world of the twenty-first century?

Fighting disease

The range of new drugs being produced every year is huge. Drug companies spend billions of pounds on research – knowing that enormous profits can be made for those who develop successful new treatments.

There are now many many different types of antibiotics that kill all sorts of bacteria – and lots of different vaccines that prevent and control diseases such as polio, measles, mumps and whooping cough.

But doctors are still *not* able to cure viral infections such as AIDS and the common cold, and cancer – although treatable – is still a major killer disease. As a result, in addition to research into cures for such illnesses, emphasis has been placed on educating people about how to *avoid* diseases like AIDS and make 'lifestyle changes' to avoid certain cancers like lung cancer.

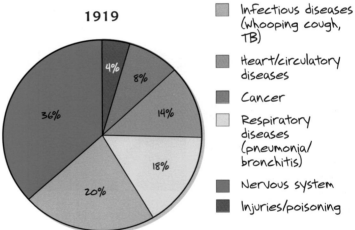

1919

- Infectious diseases (whooping cough, TB)
- Heart/circulatory diseases
- Cancer
- Respiratory diseases (pneumonia/bronchitis)
- Nervous system
- Injuries/poisoning

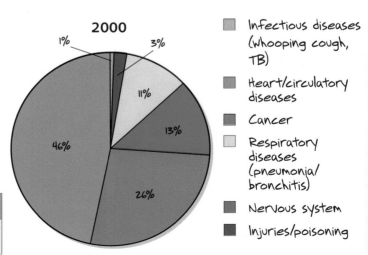

2000

- Infectious diseases (whooping cough, TB)
- Heart/circulatory diseases
- Cancer
- Respiratory diseases (pneumonia/bronchitis)
- Nervous system
- Injuries/poisoning

Source A ▶ *Causes of death in 1919 and 2000.*

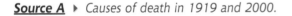

TOP EXAM TIP

Try to write your own TEN word definition for the term "alternative medicine."

148 · Medicine through time

One of the most controversial developments in the fight against disease is **genetic engineering** and **gene therapy** (see Fact box). Some of today's doctors believe that this will allow them to cure or prevent most diseases in the twenty-first century.

However, in 1999, a healthy young man who volunteered for gene therapy to cure an inherited liver complaint died of a toxic response to his treatment. Genetic engineering … and screening … though is perhaps becoming more science fact than science fiction (see **Source B**).

Source B ➤ *Based on an article in the* Daily Mail, *November 2006.*

"Angela Donovan lost her eye to a rare cancer. Her first child was born with the same illness and now she has chosen to have a 'designer baby'. The child she is expecting has been selected by genetic screening to be born free from the eye cancer that is genetic.

The eye cancer, known as retinoblastoma (RB), needs aggressive treatment and until recently, a carrier would have a 50% chance of passing it on to their children. In 2005, the Human Fertilisation and Embryology Authority granted permission to screen Angela's embryos for the eye cancer. Two embryos, without the faulty gene, were implanted using IVF.

Angela doesn't want another child to suffer what she and her son Kieran have already been through. Using this method eliminates the risk. The embryos are not modified, as many people believe. Angela's embryos were screened for this particular eye cancer and nothing else. Angela believes screening for a hereditary disease that is present at birth is different from checking for all possible illnesses or diseases.

The Human Fertilisation and Embryology Authority recently decided not to rule out screening other inheritable cancers in the future."

Hi-tech surgery

Major breakthroughs were made in the field of surgery in the twentieth century. Improved anaesthetics allowed patients to be unconscious for longer so more complicated operations could be attempted whilst better antibiotics – like penicillin – increased the success rate of difficult operations because they cut down the chances of deadly infection. When transplant surgery became more common, new drugs helped to prevent a patient's body from 'rejecting' their new organs. Keyhole surgery using small fibre-optic cameras linked to computers meant surgeons could perform operations through very small cuts whilst micro-surgery allowed them to magnify the area they were working on so they could rejoin nerves and blood vessels so that feeling can be retuned to damaged limbs.

But the development of transplant and replacement surgery goes on and on. Worn-out joints and damaged hearing are routinely replaced with artificial parts but new technological advances are enabling scientists to invent bionic body parts that could repair damage caused by accidents or disease (see **Source C**).

A new age in ultrasound

A modern use of the latest technology is the development of ultrasound. Ultrasound is very high frequency sound waves (not heard by the human ear) that are directed at the body. The sound passes through liquid and soft tissue but no solid objects. When the ultrasound hits a dense object (such as a heart valve or a bone) it bounces back as an echo. A computer is used to translate the echoes in to an image.

Ultrasound is most commonly used during pregnancy to monitor unborn babies and detect for any abnormalities. Traditionally 2-D scans have been the most common type of ultrasound – but in 2004, 4-D scans were developed which vastly improved the quality of images seen on the screen.

Ultrasound can also be used to identify heart disease and check for problems with the liver, bladder, pancreas, spleen, kidneys, uterus and ovaries.

Source C ▾ *The human body showing the latest techniques and advances in surgery and transplants.*

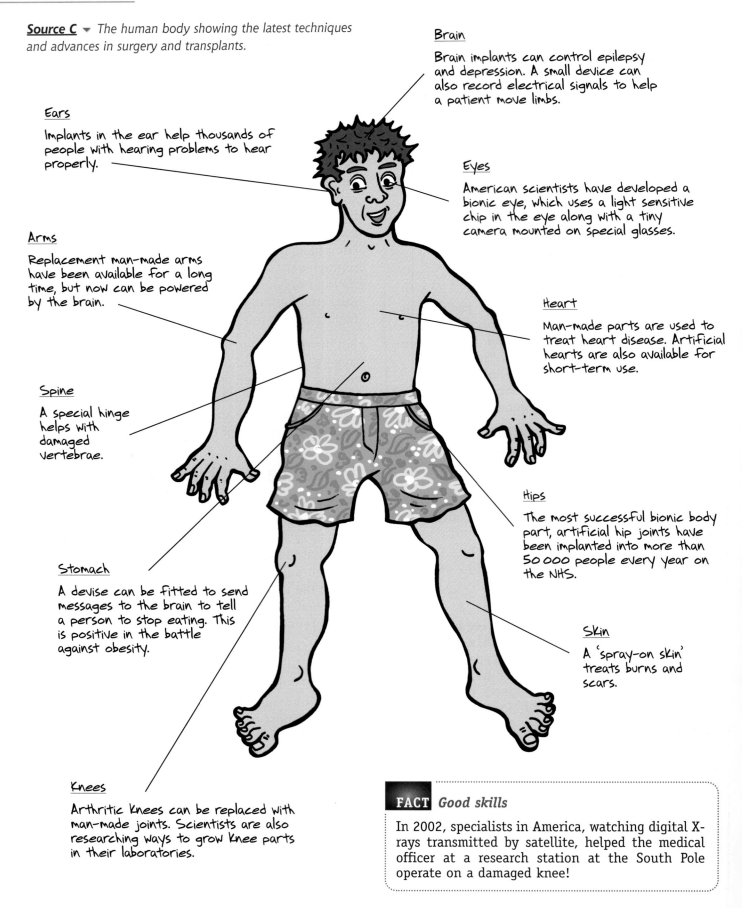

Brain

Brain implants can control epilepsy and depression. A small device can also record electrical signals to help a patient move limbs.

Ears

Implants in the ear help thousands of people with hearing problems to hear properly.

Eyes

American scientists have developed a bionic eye, which uses a light sensitive chip in the eye along with a tiny camera mounted on special glasses.

Arms

Replacement man-made arms have been available for a long time, but now can be powered by the brain.

Heart

Man-made parts are used to treat heart disease. Artificial hearts are also available for short-term use.

Spine

A special hinge helps with damaged vertebrae.

Hips

The most successful bionic body part, artificial hip joints have been implanted into more than 50 000 people every year on the NHS.

Stomach

A devise can be fitted to send messages to the brain to tell a person to stop eating. This is positive in the battle against obesity.

Skin

A 'spray-on skin' treats burns and scars.

Knees

Arthritic knees can be replaced with man-made joints. Scientists are also researching ways to grow knee parts in their laboratories.

FACT *Good skills*

In 2002, specialists in America, watching digital X-rays transmitted by satellite, helped the medical officer at a research station at the South Pole operate on a damaged knee!

'Alternative medicine'

'Alternative medicine' is the term used to describe any other way of treating an illness that doesn't rely on mainstream, doctor-dispensed scientific medicine. Those in favour of alternative medicine argue that these treatments look at the patient as a whole instead of beating a disease by finding the cause and then battering it with drugs.

Since the 1980s, alternative medicine has become more and more popular – and some of it is now available on the NHS. In fact, a recent survey indicated that one in five people in Britain have consulted alternative healers and used alternative medicines. Now even one in ten GPs are actively involved in the promotion of

alternative medicine – sometimes also called 'complementary' medicine (see **Source D**).

Some have put the increase in popularity of alternative health care down to a lack of confidence in conventional doctors and hospital care. A survey in America in the 1980s found that 2.4 million unnecessary operations were performed each year whilst in Britain in the 2000s, a number of scandals (such as that about Doctor Harold Shipman who murdered his patients and stole their money) reduced public confidence. However, an NHS survey in 2002 found that 82% of the population had visited a doctor once during the year and 90% were satisfied with their treatment.

Source D ▾ *Examples of alternative or complementary medicine.*

Aromatherapy

What? Aromatherapy is the use of essential oils from flowers, fruits, roots and leaves. The oils are inhaled or massaged into the skin.

How? The inhaled scents are said to stimulate particular parts of the brain, which promote healing while massaged oils pass into the bloodstream and can influence nervous system function, mental function and emotions.

FACT Modern aromatherapy stems from the work of French chemist Réné Gattefossé in the 1930s.

Acupuncture

What? Fine needles are placed at key points around the body. The places chosen are thought to be linked with particular needs or illnesses — but are often nowhere near the site of the pain or illness. Has been practised in China for thousands of years.

How? The needles are said to release blocked energy and balance it properly. Acupuncture allows the energy to flow again — and stimulates healing and relieves pain. It has been used as an anaesthetic during major surgery.

FACT The World Health Organization recognises 100 conditions that can be helped by acupuncture including headaches, labour pain and high blood pressure.

Some of the different types of alternative medicine

Homeopathy

What? Patients take a medicine (a plant, animal or mineral material soaked in alcohol) which causes similar symptoms to the illness they are suffering from. First practised in the late 1700s by a German doctor, Samuel Hahnemann.

How? The idea is that tiny doses of the medicine that causes similar symptoms would cure the patient by stimulating his or her natural defences. Homeo means 'like' … and homeopaths believe that 'like cures like'!

FACT Studies have shown homeopathy to be effective in treating hay fever, insomnia, depression and eczema.

Hypnotherapy

What? A therapist hypnotises the patient. When totally relaxed, the patient can be relieved of stress conditions, allergies or even physical addictions such as smoking.

How? Based on positive thinking — that the power of a patient's own mind can bring about their healing.

FACT The use of trance states to promote healing dates back to ancient times but modern hypnotherapy dates from the work of Austrian Anton Mesmer in the 1800s.

FACT *Are you qualified?*

One of the major drawbacks of alternative medicine is the lack of regulation. While conventional medicine can only be practised by a doctor who has been to medical school and passed all their exams, anyone can call themselves an alternative medicine doctor and start a business. But this is changing as the UK government begins to look into the licensing of alternative practitioners.

Source E ▾ *An extract from the report of a survey on the popularity of alternative therapies, in which 2000 people took part.*

Types of alternative therapy personally experienced	Tried by %	Satisfied?	
		Yes %	No %
Herbal medicine	12	73	18
Osteopathy	6	73	14
Massage	6	82	9
Homeopathy	4	66	16
Acupuncture	3	50	47
Chiropractic	2	68	19
Hypnotherapy	2	43	50
Psychotherapy	2	75	12

FACT *Biggest killer*

About five million people die each year from smoking, that is one in ten adults worldwide. By 2030, it is expected to kill ten million each year. Thirteen million British adults continue to smoke regularly despite advertising campaigns and evidence of its link with cancer.

FACT *The most common illness*

The most common illness in Britain is depression. Around 3.2 million people suffer and the numbers are rising. Depression costs the British economy £8 billion a year.

Positive health

In recent years, there has been a greater emphasis placed on *prevention* rather than cure – this is sometimes known as **positive health**. People are learning that regular exercise is very important for you and a good diet which avoids sugary, fatty foods can help prevent obesity and heart disease. There is also a lot of emphasis on the dangers of tobacco and the misuse of alcohol and drugs.

There has also been an increase in **screening** procedures too – this focuses on checking large numbers of people who seem to be healthy, aiming to find those who have the early signs of a serious illness like lung or breast cancer.

Source F ▾ *Schools work hard at the positive health message. Healthy eating is promoted by many schools that have dropped chocolate, fizzy drinks, burgers and chips from their menus in favour of more nutritious meals. Some Education Authorities award certificates to the healthiest schools – this one has been awarded to Castle High School in Dudley.*

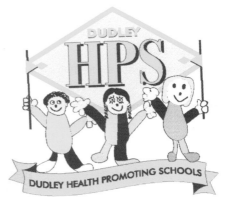

CASTLE HIGH (V.A.) SCHOOL

has made a commitment to developing health related activities

2004– 2006

 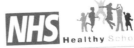 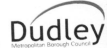

Source G ▼ *All cigarette packets carry messages warning of the dangers of smoking.*

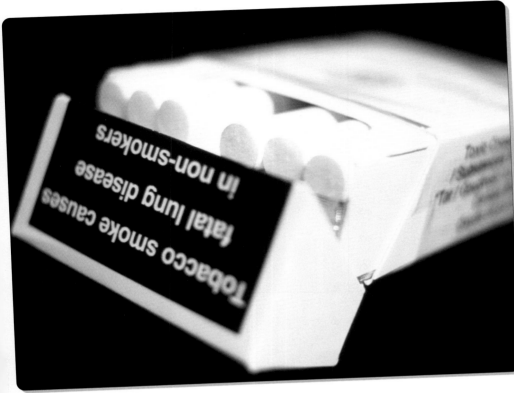

The UK and the world

Most of the medical advances studied in this book have only benefited a small minority of the world's population. People in many of the world's poorer countries die from diseases that are thought of as minor in developed countries. For example, five million children die in developing countries each year from diarrhoea, a condition easily treatable in most of the 'richer' countries of the world. So how does the UK compare to some of the richest and poorest countries in the world? Study **Sources H** to **L** to find out.

Source H ▼ *Daily food consumption.*

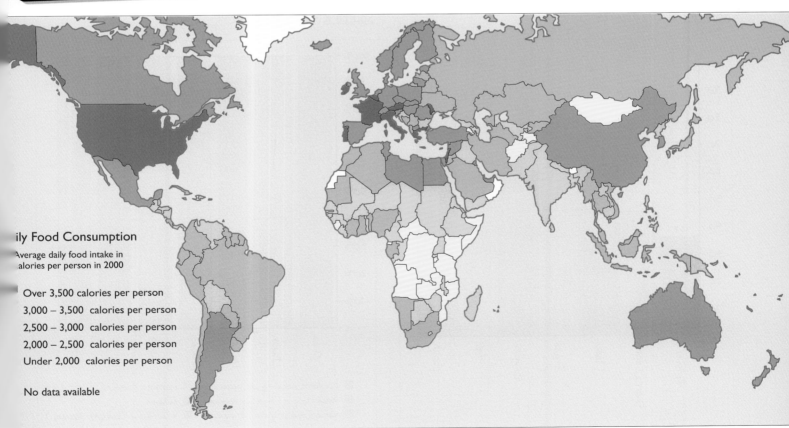

Daily Food Consumption

Average daily food intake in calories per person in 2000

Over 3,500 calories per person
3,000 – 3,500 calories per person
2,500 – 3,000 calories per person
2,000 – 2,500 calories per person
Under 2,000 calories per person

No data available

Source I ▾ *Hospital capacity – beds per 1000 people.*
Highest and lowest capacities.

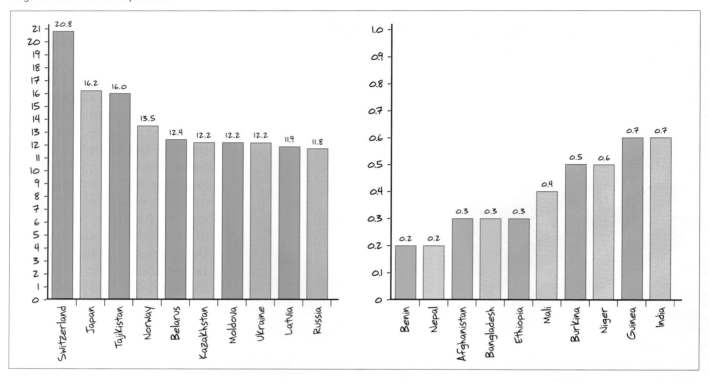

Source J ▾ *Life expectancy.*

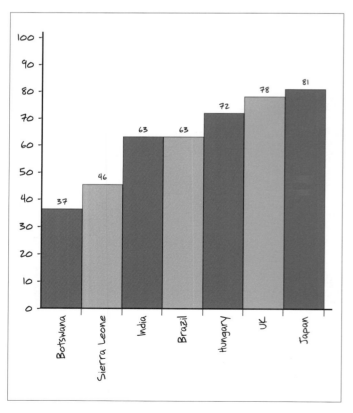

Source K ▾ *Causes of death.*

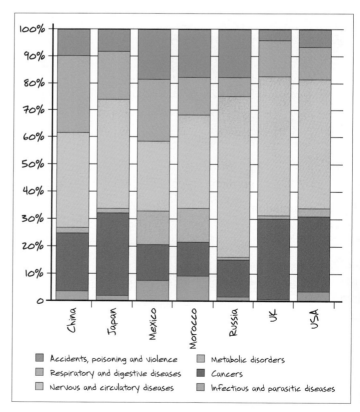

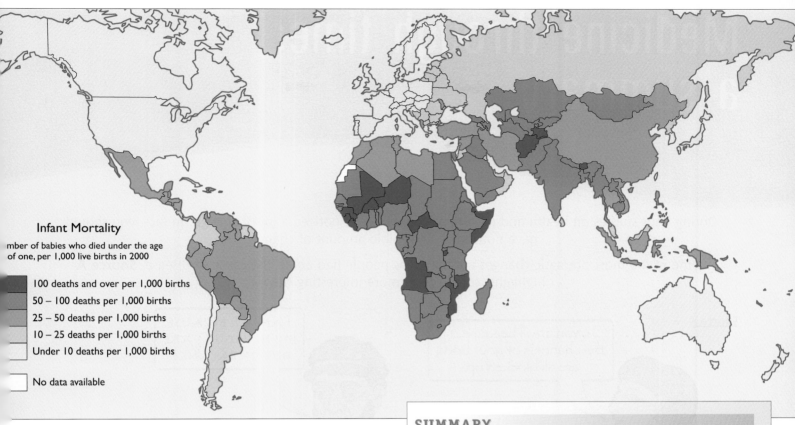

Infant Mortality

mber of babies who died under the age
of one, per 1,000 live births in 2000

- 100 deaths and over per 1,000 births
- 50 – 100 deaths per 1,000 births
- 25 – 50 deaths per 1,000 births
- 10 – 25 deaths per 1,000 births
- Under 10 deaths per 1,000 births

- No data available

<u>**Source L**</u> ▲ *Infant mortality.*

WISE UP WORDS

- screening   positive health
  genetic engineering   gene therapy

WORK

1 Look at **Source A**.

   a What have been the major changes for causes of death between 1919 and 2000?

   b Can you think of any reasons to explain these changes?

2 Look at **Source B**.

   a In your own words, explain how Angela Donovan is attempting to ensure her unborn child does not have eye cancer.

   b Genetic research is one of medicine's most controversial areas. Think about:

   i) Should we all know our own genetic make-up?

   ii) Who should have access to a person's genetic information?

SUMMARY

- Some disease (smallpox for example) has been wiped out. Effective antibiotics (like penicillin) fight infections. New killers, like AIDS, appeared – and the fight against heart disease, cancer and obesity goes on!

- Hi-tech surgery takes place, using methods such as keyhole surgery.

- The NHS provides health care for all but is underfunded and constantly under pressure.

   iii) Should everyone be forced to provide a DNA sample to be held by the government and crime prevention agencies in order to help them to solve crimes?

3 Look at **Source C**. In your opinion, which of the latest techniques is the most interesting? Give reasons for your answer.

4 **a** What is 'positive health'?

   b How has your school encouraged a more positive approach recently?

5 Look at **Sources H** to **L**. Do these sources give you any clues as to why people in Europe tend to lead healthier, longer lives than people in Africa?

Medicine through time: a summary

During your studies on health and medicine, you will have noticed a lot of change. In fact, you should have noticed an incredible amount of change.

Some of the most dramatic changes are the ideas people had about the cause of disease. **Source A** highlights some of the more interesting theories.

<u>Source A</u> ▾

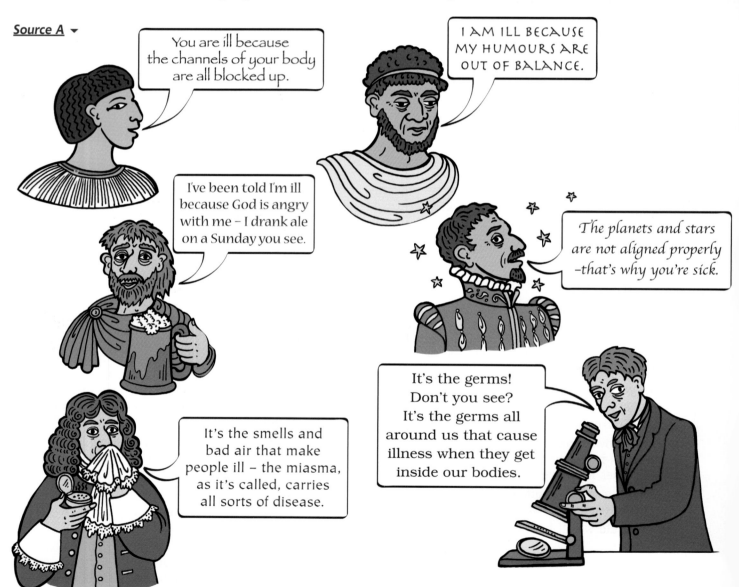

Equally as dramatic are the changing ideas and methods for treating illness and disease. **Source B** shows some of these.

Source B ▾

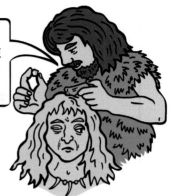

REMOVING A PIECE OF SKULL WILL RELEASE THE BAD SPIRITS THAT ARE MAKING HER ILL.

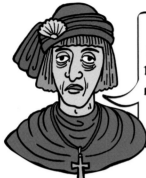

Praying to God should take away my illness. Going on a pilgrimage to a holy place will help too.

THE ONLY WAY TO GET HIM HEALTHY IS TO GET HIS HUMOURS BACK IN BALANCE. I'M BLEEDING HIM IN ORDER TO ACHIEVE THIS BALANCE – HE HAS TOO MUCH BLOOD YOU SEE!

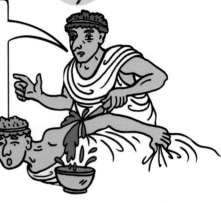

Herbal remedies have worked for hundreds of years – I will soon make a potion to help heal your wound.

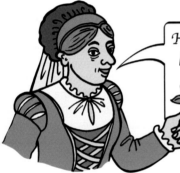

If we clean up the town, there will be less dirt. Less dirt means less smell – and less smell means less disease.

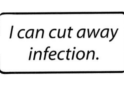

I can cut away infection.

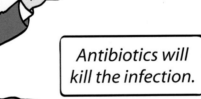

Antibiotics will kill the infection.

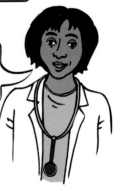

To rid myself of plague, I could rub the bottom of a dead chicken on my sores or apply the guts of a dead puppy to my forehead! Fingers crossed!

You should also have noticed a number of factors cropping up again and again during your studies. These factors are the things that have made things change – or even made things stay the same for centuries.

Take a factor like religion, for example. For centuries, the Christian Church said it was wrong to dissect human bodies for medical research and discouraged new ideas. As a result, doctors didn't perform dissection because they feared offending God. So doctors didn't learn a lot about the human body because they didn't get a chance to cut them open, look inside and study them properly. You might say then, that religion stopped medical progress and made sure it stayed the same. When the Church decided it was acceptable to dissect human bodies, doctors learned a lot very quickly. This is a very simplified, but classic, example of how a factor like religion has influenced understanding of health and medicine.

Source C pulls together some other common factors that can influence change.

<u>Source C</u> ▾

Science and technology

Advances in science and technology can improve health care dramatically. For example, from around 1200BC the invention of better quality steel instruments gave surgeons better equipment to carry out operations. And in the nineteenth century, the development of better glass meant better lenses could be used in microscopes. This meant scientists and doctors could better study the germs that cause disease.

Individual brilliance

Brilliant scientists and doctors, who were highly intelligent and full of ideas, made great discoveries that helped improve people's health. For example, Louis Pasteur devised a brilliant experiment to prove that germs caused disease.

Religion

Throughout history, religious ideas have influenced people's beliefs about the causes and cures of illness. For example, the Egyptian religious practice of mummification led to them gaining a greater understanding of the internal structure of the human body.

Chance

Sometimes luck can play its part in improving health care. For example, it was only when the battlefield surgeon, Ambroise Paré, ran out of the hot oil he usually put on wounds, that he tried his own mixture of eggs and natural oils. This mixture turned out to be a lot more effective – and a lot less painful.

Factors that can cause change

Governments

Sometimes, the government of the day makes important decisions that improve the nation's health. For example, when the British government made TB vaccination compulsory f or all schoolchildren, deaths from TB dropped dramatically.

War

Due to the high number of injuries, war often improves medical care. For example, during World War One:

* millions of wounded soldiers gave doctors the chance to try new techniques such as X-rays, blood transfusions, complex brain surgery and skin grafts;
* deep bullet wounds meant that doctors had to search harder than ever for ways to prevent infection.

Communications

Improvements in communications have been vital in the advance of health and medicine. For example, when printing was invented, new medical ideas, such as Vesalius' ideas about anatomy, could be spread quicker than ever. Even today, digital X-rays can be transmitted by satellite to help surgeons in remote locations to perform complex operations.

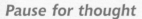

Pause for thought

Clearly, some of these factors that caused change can sometimes work together, for example, new technology, such as the printing press, allowed the individual brilliance of Vesalius' ideas to be communicated to the world.

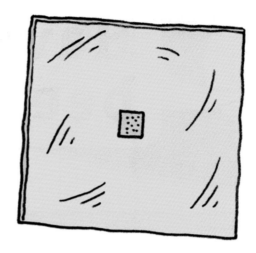

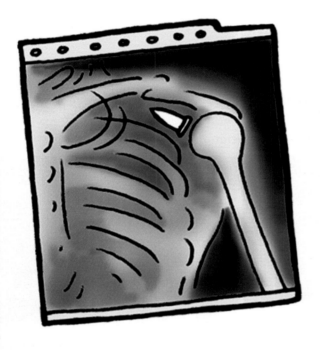

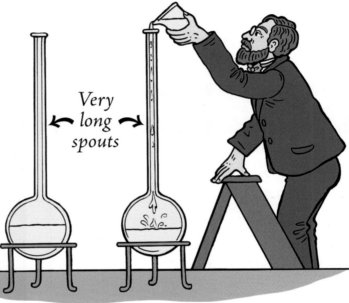

Very long spouts

WORK

1 Look at **Source A**.

   a Why were some ideas about disease believed for such a long time, even though they were wrong?

   b Do you think we know everything about disease today?

2 Look at **Source B**.

   a Which of the treatments or ideas listed are not used today?

   b Why are they no longer used?

   c Which treatments used today were not used in earlier times?

   d Why weren't they used?

3 Look at **Source C**.

   a Make your own version of **Source C**. Use pictures, diagrams and your own words. Make sure you include well-known examples of each of the factors from your studies on health and medicine.

   b Which factors do you think have been most important in the history of medicine for:
   i) causing change
   ii) preventing change?

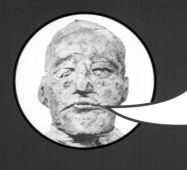

Have you been learning?

TASK 1: MEDICAL DEVELOPMENTS

Copy out and complete the following chart, which summarises medical developments in the Middle Ages and the Medical Renaissance.

Some of the boxes have been done for you.

	Middle Ages	After the Medical Renaissance
Ideas about disease	• Gods caused disease • Four humours • Ideas of Galen • Astrology • Bad air and smells	
Treatments		
Who treated illness and disease?	• Women • Doctors • Some hospitals	• Women • Doctors • More hospitals but still in a terrible condition
Interesting facts	• Not much development since Roman times • Islam preserved some of the ancient textbooks on medicine	

TASK 2: OPERATIONS

a Describe the scene in **Source A**.

b Do you think this painting is realistic?

c Why does the patient in **Source B** stand a better chance of surviving?

d What differences are there between **Source B** and a modern operation today?

▼ *Source A* *An operation in 1750.*

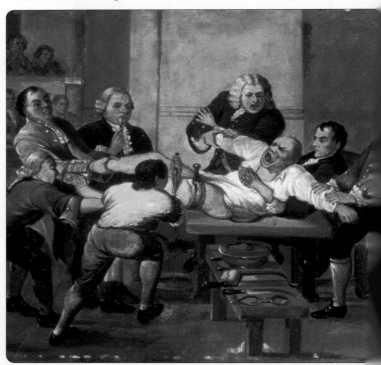

▼ *Source B* *An operation in 1900.*

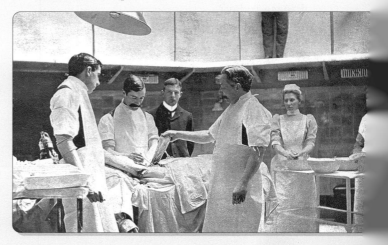

TASK 3: LATER DEVELOPMENTS

Copy out and complete the following chart, which summarises medical developments at the end of the 18th, 19th and 20th centuries.

Some of the boxes have been done for you.

	End of the 18th century	End of the 19th century	End of the 20th century
Ideas about disease	• Still belief in four humours • Knew germs existed but didn't know they caused diseases • Bad smells – 'miasma' – caused most disease		
Treat-ments	• Still attempts made to 'balance' the humours • Purging/bleeding • Only simple surgery could take place because the problems of pain, bleeding and infection hadn't been solved		
Public health		• Local councils and government took some responsibility for cleaning up the filthy towns • Average life expectancy increased but was still very low among the poor	
Individ-uals			• Alexander Fleming • Crick, Watson, Franklin

TASK 4: QUESTION TIME

Look at these genuine GCSE questions carefully. Why not try to complete them as a revision exercise? In brackets after each question, you will find the pages of this book where there is information that might refresh your memory.

- Explain the theory of spontaneous generation. (page 92)

- Explain how Pasteur proved the theory of spontaneous generation was wrong. (pages 93–95)

- 'Koch's work was more important than Pasteur's.' Explain how far you agree with this statement. (pages 93–97)

- Describe how Fleming discovered penicillin. (pages 126–131)

- Did war hinder or help the development of penicillin? (page 128)

- Was the work of Florey and Chain more important than that of Fleming? Explain your answer. (pages 127–131)

- Describe the problems that faced surgeons in the early nineteenth century. (page 108)

- Explain why some people opposed the use of antiseptics and anaesthetics. (pages 108–109)

- How far had problems in surgery been overcome by the end of the nineteenth century? (pages 110–111)

Getting your revision right

Most people experience exam nerves ... so it is perfectly natural to feel anxious when exam time approaches. But whilst a certain amount of exam stress can be used to motivate you to revise properly, it is important to keep on top of exam anxiety ... and the best way to do this is to be ORGANISED!

Before you start

Planning – Be organised, make a realistic plan you can stick to and STICK TO IT!

Be realistic – do not attempt to revise for more than 30-45 minutes at a time – break up your revision with breaks and rewards. If you give yourself a 10 minute break between two 30–45 minute sessions you will be amazed how much more you'll get done!

Support – Find a 'revision buddy' to revise with and to test you, it is often a big help.

Organise yourself – Sort out your revision environment that you are going to work in. Make sure you have everything you need – your revision books, pens, paper, stick-it notes, index cards etc. Make sure it's a quiet place where you are comfortable. Divide your work, folder or revision notes into sections that are easy to use, ordered and well structured.

Believe in yourself – You wouldn't have been given a place on the course if you didn't have the ability to do it. Therefore, if you prepare for the exams properly you should do fine, and meet your target level if not exceed it.

Keep things in perspective – The exams might seem like the most crucial thing right now, but in the grander scheme of your whole life they are only a small part.

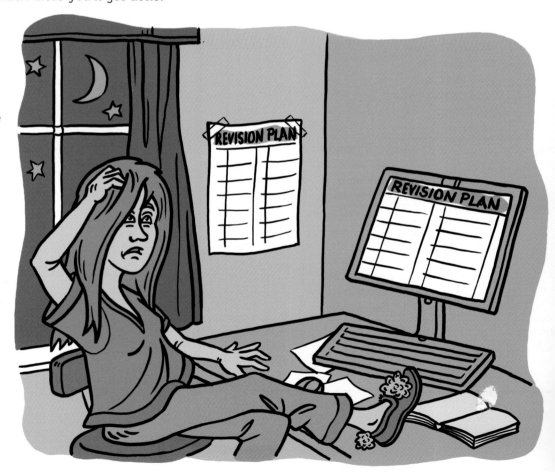

Top tips

Create an overview of what you want to revise and break each subject down into manageable chunks. Make headings and allocate each section on a monthly or weekly planner.

Set definite start and finish times for your revision sessions and have a clear goal for each session.

Build a system of regular review into your revision, checking what you know and what you don't know.

Ask your teachers for practice questions or past papers.

Practise making plans and answering questions under timed conditions.

During breaks do something completely different – listen to music, have a chocolate biscuit, make a cup of tea for example.

Use Mind Maps (see pages 120–121) for complicated topics. Use pictures and symbols that spring to your mind.

You should know how best you learn. Are you an auditory, visual or kinaesthetic learner? Make sure you use this information to help your revision.

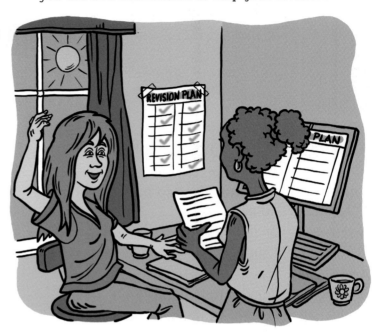

On the big day

Don't work all through the night, get an early night instead.

Make sure you know where and when the exam is and leave plenty of time to get there.

Make sure you have all your equipment in advance ... and spare pens!

Avoid too much nicotine and caffeine. Water is best – if you are 5% dehydrated, then your concentration drops 20%.

Don't listen to people who might try to wind you up about what might come up in the exam – they don't know any more than you!

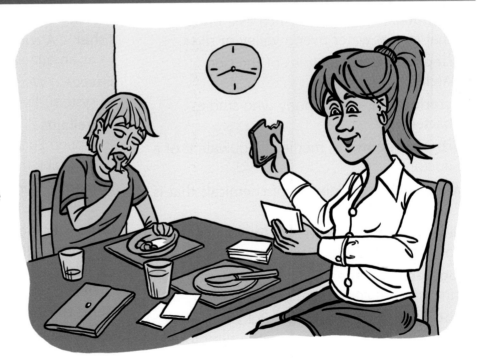

And finally, when you come out of your exam don't listen to what other people tell you *they* have written, they might not be right. This could knock your confidence, especially if you have another paper to go!

Glossary

Amputation   The removal of a limb or part of a limb by surgery.

Anaesthetic   A drug given to make a person insensitive to pain.

Anatomy   The science of understanding the structure of the body.

Antibiotics   A group of drugs used to treat infections, for example penicillin.

Antiseptic   Chemicals used to destroy germs and prevent infection.

Apothecary   A chemist or pharmacist.

Aqueducts   A structure (such as a bridge) that carries water over a valley or river.

Asclepeia   Greek temples of the God Asclepius.

Bacteriologist   Somebody who studies bacteria.

Barber-surgeon   A medieval equivalent of a doctor.

Barium meal   A mixture of chemicals that is opaque to X-rays.

Bill of mortality   A weekly list of the causes of death in a particular place.

Bloodletting   The release of a patient's blood in order to 'cure' them.

Bubonic   A type of plague. Boils under the arms (buboes) were one of the symptoms.

Cautery   A red-hot iron used to cauterise (seal) a wound.

Chloroform   An anaesthetic liquid whose vapour makes a person unconscious.

Contagion   The passing of disease from one person to another.

Dissection   Cutting up and examination of a body.

DNA   Deoxyribonucleic acid, the molecule that genes are made from.

Embalmers   Men who treated (embalmed) dead bodies to preserve them.

Epidemics   An outbreak of disease that affects a large number of people.

Ether   A colourless sweet-smelling liquid used as an anaesthetic.

Faeces   Waste material from the digestive system. Poo in other words!

Flagellants   A group of people who walked around Europe during the Black Death whipping themselves as penance for man's sins.

Forceps   Surgical instrument used in childbirth.

Gene   Part of the nucleus of a cell that determines how our bodies look and function. Genes are passed from parents to their children.

Gene therapy   Involves inserting genes into somebody's cells to treat a disease.

Genetic engineering   The investigation of genes and how they can be changed to make the body work better.

Germ Theory   The theory that germs cause disease.

Hieroglyphics   A form of writing using picture symbols, as used in Ancient Egypt.

Human Genome Project   A project to de-code and identify human genes.

Infant mortality   The number of children who die before their first birthday.

Inoculation   Putting a low dose of a disease into the body to help it fight against a more serious attack of the same disease.

IVF treatment   A technique where egg cells are fertilised outside the mother's body. *In vitro* means *in glass* and refers to the test tube used.

Laissez faire   The belief that governments should not interfere in people's lives.

Laxatives   A medicine that makes a person empty their bowels.

Leeches   A blood-sucking worm used to drain blood.

Ligature   A thread used to tie a blood vessel during anoperation.

Magic bullet   Something that could kill a disease without hurting the patient.

Miasma   Smells from rotting material that were believed to cause and spread disease.

Mummification   An ancient way of preserving the body, common in ancient Egypt.

Papyrus   Early 'paper' made from a plant.

Pneumonia   The inflammation of the lungs due to an infection.

Positive health   The focus on the prevention of illness and disease rather than cure.

Prehistoric   The period before the writing of history begins.

Preventive medicine   Ways of preventing illness from starting.

Public health   The well-being of the whole community.

Purging   The act of taking medicine that makes you vomit.

Quacks   People who falsely claim to have medical ability and sell 'cure-all' potions and medicine.

Radiotherapy   The treatment of disease by a form of radiation.

Screening   Checking for the presence of a disease.

Spontaneous generation   The idea that living things can come into existence by themselves, rather than being born and so on.

Sterilise   To destroy all germs from surfaces or surgical instruments.

Theory of the four humours   The belief that the body contains four liquids – blood, phlegm, yellow bile and black bile. The ancient Greeks and others after them believed that health depended on having the right amounts of these humours in the body.

Trepanning   The drilling of a hole in the skull.

Ultrasound scan   A scan using sound or vibrations with an ultrasonic frequency. Used in medical imaging, especially during pregnancy to examine the fetus.

Vaccination   The injection into the body of weakened germs to give the body resistance against disease.

Welfare state   A system by which the government looks after the well-being of the nation, particularly those who cannot help themselves, such as the old, children, the sick, unemployed and so on.

Witch doctor   Someone who tries to cure illness by magic, especially conmen in prehistoric tribes.

X-ray   An image made by the effect of X-rays on a photographic plate.

Index